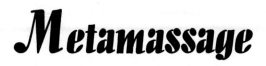

Metamassage

by **PYRRHA MALOUF**

Illustrations by Sandra Cummings

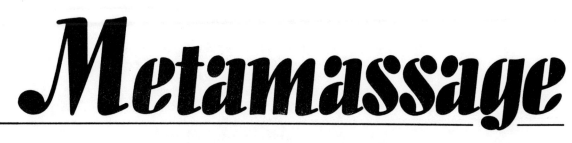

Metamassage

HOW TO MASSAGE YOUR WAY TO A BEAUTIFUL COMPLEXION—ALL OVER

PRIAM BOOKS

ARBOR HOUSE
NEW YORK

Library of Congress Catalogue Card Number: 83-70488

ISBN: 0-87795-472-0

Manufactured in the United States of America

10 9 8 7 6 5 4 3 2 1

This book is printed on acid free paper. The paper in this book meets the guidelines for permanence and durability of the Committee on Production Guidelines for Book Longevity of the Council on Library Resources.

To my mother, who bore me and who has borne with me ever since

Acknowledgments

Thank you and abundant blessings to the following people who have contributed to the writing of this book: Totty Ames, Carol Ardman, Cheryl Ashley, Fran Attaway and Larry Becker, Zackory, Joshua and Nodiah Brent, Helen Gurley Brown, Andrea Charman, Del Coleman, Stan Corwin, Sudy Dostal, Carolyn Robinson Gulliland, Jeff Justice, Jody Morris, Raquel Ruben, Mallen De Santis, Inga Schiller, Frank Tingue, Sarah Uman, Kenneth Woods. I would also like to thank all my many friends and family, especially my mother and father, for their love, advice and continued support.

Contents

PREFACE   13

YOUR FACE   27

Introduction to METAMASSAGE   29

The Mental Preparation   35

Muscles and Cells   38

What You Need   42

The Preliminaries   46

The Routine   49

Post METAMASSAGE   63

If You Have Had Cosmetic Surgery   72

Sunbathing and METAMASSAGE   75

Sleeping and Skin Care   77

Masks   81

Your Hair   86

YOUR BODY   97

Introduction to Body Ritual and Routine   99

Muscles, Nerves and Glands   102

Ames Body Alignment   104

The Bath   114

METAMASSAGE as a Lifetime Discipline   141

Other Things I Do   144

Care Enough   149

Bibliography   153

Saints and kings, prophets and dervishes, all bow down before beauty, descending from the unknown world.

We love beauty because it is not merely of this Earth, beauty in the human being is a reflection of celestial beauty itself.

—*Secret Garden,*
Sufi writings of the 13th century

The real sin against life is to abuse and destroy beauty, even one's own—even more, one's own, for that has been put in our care and we are responsible for its well-being.

—*Ship of Fools,*
Katherine Anne Porter

I have nothing against aging, I just never wanted to look or feel old. To counteract the phenomenon of advancing age, except for brief forays into studied dissipation, hot dogs and candy bars, I have watched my eating habits. But eating sensibly, by itself, does not stop one from looking older. Even "good genes" are not the total answer. Exercise can keep you looking trim, but won't do a thing for rough, wrinkled or blemished skin.

By age thirty one begins to assess and tally one's successes and failures in life. People who have not scored themselves high usually decide that this is the time to "do something about it." Some go back to college to explore new fields, others turn to philosophy and religion. Still others become enmeshed in physical activities and clubs, if for no other reason than to "belong" with their fellow humans. Those who don't have children and want them feel an urgency to procreate. Most want to do something, *anything*, that makes them feel the world is not passing them by...and that they're not being out-distanced by age.

One thing we *can* do to make our lives better at any age and reap long-term benefits is replace those habits that don't give us satisfaction. I have devised a technique which allows me to enjoy life by feeling and looking as good as possible as I advance in age.

At the top of my priorities is making the most of what I have to work with, and continuing to learn how to apply a few well-chosen principles toward greater wisdom and understanding. Life presents a grand opportunity for joyous experiences that I do not want to miss because of ignorance, or because I'm too old to see or enjoy them anymore. I choose to remain young in heart and body and only to grow old in soul. From this cognition META-MASSAGE was born, raised and grew. It is mine and yours—and it works!

Starting from the Teenage Years

It is interesting that *Webster's New Collegiate Dictionary* includes the following definition of what was previously meant by "teen"—misery, affliction. These tumultuous years between thirteen and nineteen are full of changes. Physiological, psychological, psychic, hormonal and glandular changes are a source of much confusion for the teenager. I remember wondering if I had any control over my faculties whatsoever. METAMASSAGE was beginning to take shape in my mind during this period of my life. I really strived to outdistance bad skin, greasy hair, a body whose appendages didn't seem to match, and a chronic unwelcome lump in my throat that wouldn't leave due to my insecurity. I sought refuge in books and magazines on beauty. Over the years, through trial and error and a lot of experimentation, this simple formula for self-care was devised, helping me cross the Rubicon of those awkward times.

You, too, are a person concerned about yourself and your appearance or you wouldn't be thumbing through this book. How long did it take you to walk into a bookstore and head for the beauty section? After trying how many methods of skin care, experimentation with cosmetics and trips to the dermatologist did you finally decide to see what the experts who write books could tell you? How many books did you look through before picking up this one? If the answer is several, I don't blame you. I, too, have never missed a chance to read anything I can on beauty and self-improvement—and this motivation was the starting point of my search for lovely skin and a beautiful complexion. But your search can be, as mine was, time consuming and confusing, given the often contradictory information we read about the care and treatment of our skin.

METAMASSAGE was developed through a great deal of reading, studying, observation and experimentation. From a very early age I devoured anything I could to help me with my "problem" teenage skin, trying every suggestion I chanced upon. Some worked temporarily, while others did nothing at all. But I continued to experiment, confident that there had to be a way to improve on a somewhat less than perfect complexion.

It wasn't until I made my way to Hollywood and worked for the Helene Segar Cosmetic Company that the bits and pieces of knowledge I'd accumulated began to come into focus for me. Helene Segar offered an excellent program in which she trained her beauty consultants, like myself, to sell cosmetics. The Segar Company offered cleansing aids and make-up, with an emphasis on make-up. I saw several women daily and gained a vast knowledge of the skin woes—some major and some not so major—that plague women. The experience proved to be an invaluable one, teaching me that even though no two women are alike, there is a similarity in the problems that spoil a woman's complexion. Though at the time I had no solution for those women, I was determined to find a way to help them improve on what they had to work with.

Soon I graduated from door-to-door cosmetic sales to the "House of Galenti." Cora Galenti, a fascinating woman of indeterminate age, manufactured a line of products in the same building which housed her skin-peeling salon. The emphasis in the House of Galenti was initially on skin care, but I learned even more from watching Miss Galenti manufacture her creams and cleansers. It was through her that I came to believe that with a lot of discipline and care one never had to look old. One look at her and you became a believer! My job at the House of Galenti was to instruct the ladies on how to apply the creams and remove them after their special treatments. The clients were supposed to come back every few weeks so that Miss Galenti could check their progress. I was given another opportunity to learn about skin as she checked to see who was preserving herself "according to Galenti." It was plain to see who was maintaining their newfound beauty and who was not. I could not have had a more valuable apprenticeship. I don't know what ever became of Cora Galenti, but I will be eternally grateful to her for adding to my knowledge and philosophy of beauty.

During this time I also became interested in yoga. There is an old proverb which states that "when the student is ready, the master appears . . ." In my case it came true, as I'd heard of a respected yogi teaching in Hollywood. It was my belief that, while improving my appearance was important, I should also attain discipline of the inner self. The wonderful man who I encountered, Ivan Markoff, sensed my sincere desire to learn about myself and accepted me as a student.

My association with him lasted 22 years until my beautiful guru died in Hawaii in 1969. I was shattered for several years afterward but I had learned so much from him about inner discipline that the same principles I learned those many years ago still sustain me now. METAMASSAGE was evolving through more than just learning about skin care.

It was during this time that I married a musician, and my lifestyle changed abruptly. We traveled on the road a lot, which can be pretty grueling, and it took a great deal of discipline to maintain my mind and body. I remember how the band's lead singer would look at me in amazement every morning and comment on how wonderful I looked. She queried me about what my secret was. At this time I was still referring to METAMASSAGE as "doing my face." This was a misnomer at best. I should have been calling it "doing my face and neck," the neck being as important as the face. I told her about my method of skin care which, by this time, was past the incubation stage and beginning to take shape as a special technique from which I could attain lasting results.

As my marriage disintegrated, my career in the acting field began to blossom. Soon I was going to interviews and getting jobs in movies, television and theater in Los Angeles. This was one of the greatest periods of my life since I loved the glamour and glamorous people. It was very hard work, but the fact that I was getting paid a lot of money to do something I enjoyed made it seem almost too good to be true. Though my life had taken a different direction, I was still interested in learning everything I could from the make-up people, hairdressers and costumers I had the opportunity to work with. The make-up people could hardly apply my make-up, I was so full of questions. It was the same with the hairdressers and costume designers.

But all that make-up takes its toll after years of working under hot, bright lights. Many a complexion has been permanently scarred because years ago make-up had a lead and mercury base, much the same as during Elizabeth I's reign. If you were smart you removed the heavy make-up immediately, but a lot of people didn't know how to do that correctly. There used to be a lot of skin problems in the entertainment industry. Fortunately the Food and Drug Administration put stringent controls on make-up components and today the trend in all the cosmetic houses is toward using natural ingredients. Even with today's advanced technology, though, if one is not careful to remove cosmetics thoroughly (particularly at night when the skin has gained a veneer of pollutants and grime) the pores become clogged and skin problems multiply.

I am not against make-up or enhancing one's bone structure with cosmetics. I *am* against the tawdry practice of leaving skin care to chance or half-hearted practices. Having beautiful, smooth skin underneath cosmetics augments their purpose and effectiveness. I don't know what I'd do without the choice of all the wonderful magical potions at my disposal. What a pleasure it is to be able to change one's mood and countenance with a variety of products. But I want to feel as confident about my looks *without* these helpmates as I do *with* them.

There are scores of books on the application of make-up. With a bit of skill amazing effects can be created. But this is not a book on how to paint portraits on our faces. My concern is about the canvas beneath the portrait.

I am fortunate to have taught METAMASSAGE to such beautiful women as film stars Esther Williams, Audrey Totter and Jill St. John, and to author and *Cosmopolitan* editor Helen Gurley Brown. Although I had toyed with the idea of writing a book on METAMASSAGE, Helen Gurley Brown inspired my efforts by asking me to write an article for *Cosmopolitan*. We had first met in Los Angeles in the early sixties. Having remarried, I had just completed my fourth pregnancy in five years. Helen had recently written the highly successful *Sex and the Single Girl,* and was (and still is) married to motion picture executive David Brown. By this time my career had shifted from film to home. I was struggling along raising three children (the second pregnancy ended in a miscarriage), entertaining often and missing my film career something fierce. Helen was beginning to achieve the recognition she rightfully deserved. Around this time I moved to Morocco; Helen became editor of *Cosmopolitan* and we lost touch with each other for many years. Usually I would pass through Los Angeles or New York City en route to and from Europe, and just miss Helen on either coast, as she was traveling extensively also. We spoke on the phone but were never able to mesh schedules in order to see each other. On one of those jaunts, though, our timing coincided and we had a delightful, happy reunion. I thought she was as lovely as ever and she thought I looked great too. After we'd had a chance to catch up on what we each had been doing for the past several years, Helen admired the fact that I had not changed much in appearance and asked how I kept looking so young. I explained METAMASSAGE to her and she was interested enough in the technique to set up a meeting with Mallen De Santis, the beauty editor of *Cosmopolitan*. The two of them invited me to write an article for the magazine, which I did, that was published in 1978. Subsequently another article on the bathing technique was published in 1980, and the seed of expanding the articles into a book was planted.

The wonderful thing about remaining young looking is that people whom you haven't seen for a long time are always asking you what your secret is. I suppose my basic secret is trying to keep in step with the world and a step ahead of myself. I also am a great experimenter. Though the many beauty formulas you'll find in METAMASSAGE are all tried and true, I continue to look for new ones, trying different facial exercises, body exercises, creams, lotions, herbs, vitamins...everything. But the METAMASSAGE technique is one thing I'll always stick to. Nothing has worked as well for me and I'll never give it up.

In traveling around the world I've observed that people everywhere have skin problems that make them look old, but I refuse to let my skin reveal my true age. No matter what their particular customs are or their methods of skin care, all have the same problems of skin eruptions, blackheads and whiteheads, large pores and multitudinous lines. No one is happy with these skin problems. METAMASSAGE helps you to have beautiful skin by teaching you how to cleanse thoroughly, increase circulation, regenerate energy and smooth lines and creases. I've taught my method in the Middle East, Europe, India, Mexico, the West Indies and America, all with the same wonderful results.

Helena Rubinstein wrote in her book, *My Life for Beauty,* "There are no ugly women, only lazy ones." For META-MASSAGE to work for you, you must stop being lazy about yourself, quit indulging in wishful thinking and *act.* Knowledge and application of that knowledge are what count. The wonderful thing about life is that it's never too late to drop a bad habit or to acquire a beneficial new one. I, too, must work to keep myself motivated. It's fun to be lazy. I can easily get used to treading the path of least resistance. But as an acquaintance of mine once said, "You have to be disciplined in order to be flexible." And you have to be flexible to keep yourself feeling and looking young.

The METAMASSAGE routine you're about to learn helps you to work on yourself from the *internal,* through relaxation and proper breathing, to the *external,* through self-massage. Every facet of METAMASSAGE has been thought out and experimented upon over a period of many years. There are no short cuts to lasting beauty, though the magazines may tell you otherwise. METAMASSAGE is as close to a short cut as you'll come. Perhaps you're thinking you're too busy with your career or family and that, along with your other self-improvement activities, you won't have time for this one, too. The techniques in this book will not only cut down on time spent on many of your superfluous, "quickie" attempts to increase your natural beauty, but will reward you with the long-term benefits of beautiful, silky, clear skin. Activate your body to do its inherent work by Metamassaging daily, and through this regenerative cleansing method you can and will thwart the signs of aging. Father Time needn't be your dad—or mine!

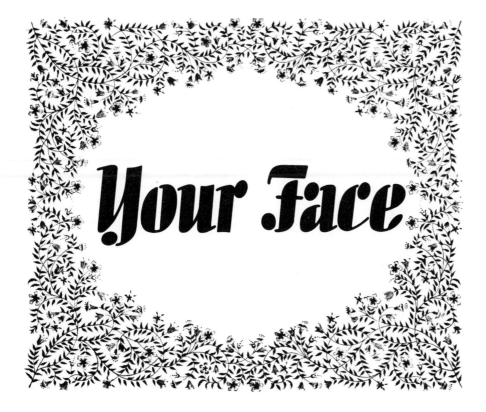

INTRODUCTION TO METAMASSAGE

met'a (Greek) A prefix
meaning in general,
along with—

1. a Posteriority or
succession, as in
metagenesis;
   b Change;
transportation;
transfer as in
metamorphosis;
   c (From
metaphysics)
Beyond,
transcending,
higher.

mas-sage', n.
(French) A method of
treating the body for
remedial or hygienic
purposes, consisting
of rubbing, stroking,
kneading, tapping,
etc., with the hand or
an instrument.

METAMASSAGE is a practical and efficient method of self-massage that prevents signs of the aging process. Dead cells, sagging muscles and unbecoming skin color due to faulty circulation—the primary reasons for poor skin—can be eliminated with my method of skin care.

METAMASSAGE works to eliminate blemishes and smooth wrinkles caused by incorrect skin cleansing habits. Skin renewal will be evident the first time this technique is applied. Each of us generates our own potent energy force; in using the concept behind META-MASSAGE—Energy Replacement Therapy—you will be learning to *treat* rather than camouflage your skin problems. Approximately one hour a day for two weeks will set you on a course toward beautiful skin for the rest of your life. Not only will your attitude toward yourself change as a result of your clear, smooth complexion, you will gain new confidence as you get in tune with your body.

Energy Replacement Therapy

Place your palms two inches from your face—remain still and quiet. You will feel the energy you generate, your own potent force.

It is this energy that, through self-massage, you will learn to direct back to yourself to replenish what's been used. Think of your entire body as a

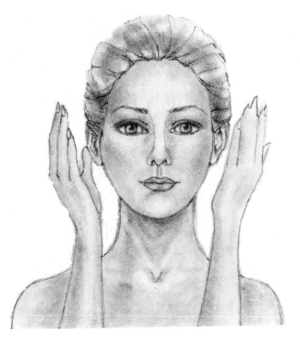

potent energy force. By using this energy and making the effort to care for your skin, you'll help your body to do its natural work through cell renewal. There is no reason to have bad skin if you are willing to work against that possibility.

Starting from the Inside Out

One-third of the toxins in your body are released through the skin by perspiration. For this reason METAMASSAGE is important in helping the body to slough off dead cells that would otherwise clog the pores. Another third of the toxins are released through the excretory channels. Therefore, a beneficial, healthful diet is most important. The other third of the poisons in the body are eliminated through the respiratory system. So we must learn to breathe deeply and fully.

The moment you feel the need to urinate or move your bowels, *do it*. Even movie stars and heads of state have been known to eliminate, so don't be embarrassed about bodily functions. There is no sense in keeping impurities inside and then having to fret over them on the outside. Body chemistry changes almost every seven years. Let your body teach you how to adapt to these changes for optimum health and a sense of well-being. Look at your body, be aware of it and listen to it. If you give all your time and energy to everyone else, you'll have none for yourself. With just a bit of organization it really doesn't take much time at all to care for yourself. But what rewards!

If you are on a special diet, adhere to it. But be aware that we are all unique individuals sharing certain common tendencies. Each of us requires a personalized diet; just as vitamin and mineral supplements are personalized for problem skin and scars, a balance of vitamins A and E is particularly valuable. As our body chemistry changes so do its needs. You will find helpful and fascinating reading in the vitamin method of Adele Davis. I suggest her book, *Let's Eat Right to Keep Fit* (New American Library). Other recommended reading is any of George Ohsawa's books on macrobiotics, *Healing Ourselves*, by Naboru Muramoto, Avon Books, and any or all books by nutritionist Bernard Jensen, available at health food stores or by writing to BER-NARD JENSEN PRODUCTS, P.O. Box 8, Solana Beach, California 92075, and Richard France's *Healing Naturally* (Amazing Books, Box 9002–334, Boulder, Colorado 80301). Arnold Ehret has written several books on fasting, a regime for which one *must* prepare. At the health food store you will see books on herbs, cell salts and proper cooking methods. Get interested in your well-being and peruse this section. They're talking about *you, me, us.* Through the regenerative cleansing method, inside and out, you will look better, feel fit and yes . . . even now . . . reverse the aging process. Make time your ally.

THE MENTAL PREPARATION

Relax

Before you begin METAMASSAGE, picture to yourself some relaxing scene or concentrate on a pleasant thought and absorb the serenity it represents to you. Maybe you love the seashore. Picture the last time you walked on a white sandy beach, and try to recapture the peacefulness of that moment. Better yet, imagine doing it now! Try to relax your mind and facial muscles. Breathe deeply and keep this picture in mind while METAMASSAGING your face.

Now exhale and then breathe in, through the nose, slowly holding the breath for three seconds. Exhale forcibly through the mouth. Do this cleansing breath three times. At the end of the last breath drop your chin to the chest and slowly roll the head around three times to the right and then three times to the left, breathing gently all the while. Be sure the spine is straight and the head level. Any tension in the neck or shoulders will have disappeared; your mind will be serene and your body alert but relaxed.

Discipline Yourself

Before long, the self-discipline META-MASSAGE requires will become a part of your life and will make a happier you. You will have mastered a new technique and your efforts will be evident to all with whom you come in contact.

I suggest you carry out METAMASSAGE without looking into a mirror. You should become intimately acquainted with your bone structure, skin texture and your relaxed self. Once you've disciplined yourself to METAMASSAGE daily, you'll find that it can be carried out in all settings: in the dark, on a train, plane, car, sitting in bed watching television or listening to music. There is no excuse for neglecting your all-important skin.

Think Positively

It is your willpower, concentration and concern that help you to translate internal thoughts and desires into external action. If you really want a more beautiful complexion, it is possible if you will make the effort. I do not suggest camouflaging skin faults but rather, correcting them with META-MASSAGE. None of us is ugly, just neglected. Start your regime now and you will not only feel pretty, you'll *be* pretty. The results from the very first facial treatment with METAMASSAGE will astound you!

Have you noticed the glow, the stimulated sensation that results from physical exercise? In the same way METAMASSAGE produces a feeling of confidence and well-being, resulting from positive action. The response from your skin will be evident each time you METAMASSAGE, so begin now, *tonight*, toward a more lustrous, radiant you.

......
MUSCLES AND CELLS

There are twenty-one pairs of voluntary facial muscles and one solitary muscle encircling the lips. These muscles are under the control of your will. There are also small groups of involuntary muscles that modify the expression to a slight extent.

Lack of muscle tone causes the skin to lose elasticity. My method of META-MASSAGE will improve your circulation and result in toned muscle fibers. For some women who neglect the forty-three facial muscles face lifts are necessary because these fibers have lost their effectiveness. If you make META-MASSAGE part of your daily routine, though, a face lift will never be necessary.

Lines and wrinkles are not always related to advanced age. You may have facial lines at forty, thirty or even twenty. A healthy skin should be moist, pliable, smooth-textured and blemish-free. Skin, the largest organ of the body, is composed of the *epidermis* (the outer layer) and the *dermis* (the inner layer). Here millions of cells are continually

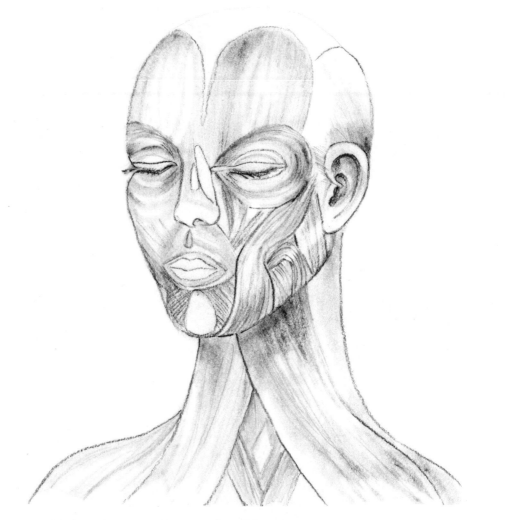

shed and renewed approximately every
two weeks. They must be nourished
and helped in their effort to slough off

so that the healthy new cells may easily travel from the inner layer to the outer layer of the skin. The dead cells quite naturally collect on the skin surface unless they are properly removed. METAMASSAGE removes these dead cells and compensates for the resulting decrease of moisture in the skin.

The effort you make to improve your appearance, your attitude about everything past and present and how much you care about your outward appearance will be reflected in METAMAS-

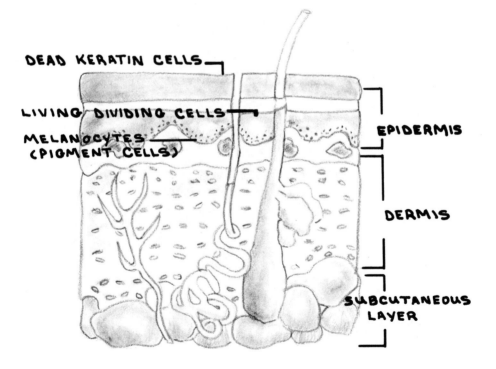

DEAD KERATIN CELLS

LIVING DIVIDING CELLS

MELANOCYTES (PIGMENT CELLS)

EPIDERMIS

DERMIS

SUBCUTANEOUS LAYER

SAGE. Everything and everyone responds to care.

Since the beginning of time women have fought a battle against showing their age. In reality they have in their hands tremendous radiating energy with which to rejuvenate themselves. Remember, you have only to place your palm two inches from your face and hold it there to feel your innate energy. You are dispensing this energy all the time to children, husbands, lovers, friends and associates, but putting little of this potent force back into yourself.

We go to masseuses and have facials in salons thinking that others must give us relaxation and replace natural energy for us. However, our personal resources are a great force. By consistent application of METAMASSAGE you will feel fresh and look radiantly alive. Drinking, smoking, partying, lack of sleep and carousing are not the real enemies. You know your limitations, so it is your lack of discipline and positive application of energy which leave tell-tale marks of age on you. Establish the habit of reserving 30 minutes to an hour a day for your improvement regime and you will achieve the same astounding results I and others have.

WHAT YOU NEED

Eye make-up remover. There are many brands of eye make-up remover in many different forms on the market. Some people are allergic to the ingredients, though. Shop around until you find a brand that suits you. Baby oil applied with a cotton pad works well for many women.

Cleansing cream, astringent or toner (if your skin is dry or sensitive) and moisturizer. You need not use the most expensive cleansing creams, astringents, toners or moisturizers. The expense of many of these products lies in their perfumes and in packaging. My beauty aids cost me approximately $10.00 a month. Often I use Pond's Cold Cream, occasionally switching to another brand. Our bodies quickly adapt and get used to a product, thus minimizing its effectiveness. Rarely do I use any brand of astringent more than once before switching to another. Then I'll return to the previous kind after a time. There are many good astringents on the market and I adore trying new products. The moisturizer that I've found works best for my skin is *"2nd Debut,"* distributed by Beecham of Clifton, N.J. It is available in two strengths, the pink being the stronger one and my favorite. About once a week I'll use a moisturizer over my *entire* face and neck. I didn't start using a moisturizer, except for around my eyes and on my neck, until I was over fifty years old. To saturate the skin with heavy emollients every day or night causes the fat glands to become overactive and the pores to become clogged, thus creating skin problems such as blackheads and pimples. We are all individual and perhaps your skin can "take" a moisturizer seven days a week, but it isn't really necessary *and can do more harm than good.*

Experiment with the well-known, less expensive brands of creams and read labels and other information included by their manufacturers. Don't be afraid to try different products until you find one that particularly suits you. Check also in the health food stores' cosmetic sections for introductory offers or specially discounted items. There is a whole new world of creams containing amino acids, vitamins A and E, and collagen, which is the material that holds cells together in your body. Although the vast array of products on the market can be mind-boggling and new ones come out every day, enjoy looking and learning and experimenting to find those products that seem to have been created just for your skin.

Cotton pads and three or even four white towels. Rexall and other drugstores manufacture their own brand of cotton pads which are usually rather inexpensive. It is well worth investing in three or four white towels, even if you already have some, to use on your face alone. You must wash them often,

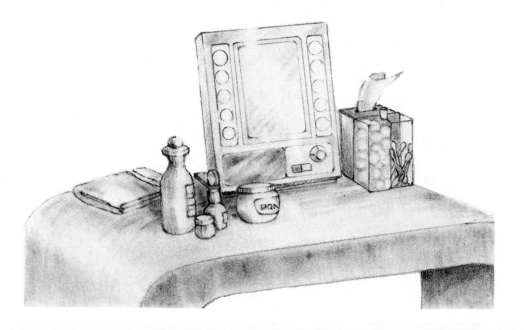

of course, using hot water, a strong detergent and bleach. Always wash them separately from the rest of your laundry.

Collect all of the things you'll need before you begin the program, and *don't let anyone else use them*—bacteria are easily transmitted in this way.

THE PRELIMINARIES

Why You Should METAMASSAGE at Night

METAMASSAGE is more effective when done at night before retiring. That way you will be cleansing your skin of the day's make-up and air pollution and your pores will not be clogged by their residue, reducing the likelihood of skin eruptions, blackheads and enlarged pores. Lines and creases will be smoothed more rapidly as the muscles of the face and neck are relaxed from the routine and you sleep more restfully.

During the first two weeks you may want to treat your face and neck both morning and night. Whether you have dry or oily skin or a combination of both, in a short time you will develop a balanced, uniform, soft, smooth-textured skin with smaller pores and a transluscent glow. METAMASSAGE has the immediate therapeutic effect of firming the facial muscles while toning the skin and defying the constant pull of gravity at the same time. Thirty minutes on a slant board once a day strengthens one's battle against the force of gravity.

Mirror Routine

Get a good quality magnifying mirror and study your face. Pay attention to the texture, pores, serious lines and potential wrinkles. With the back of your index finger stroke your cheek upward to judge the firmness of the skin. Look carefully at your skin like this once a week and you'll be amazed with the progress you're making.

Hands

Before you begin to METAMASSAGE, wash your hands. Now put cleansing cream on your hands and wrists. Lavishly stroke them ten to twenty times with the cream. Do not neglect the backs of your hands. The skin is thin here and shows age more quickly due to the many chores we use hands for and their constant exposure to soap, housework cleansers and water. I massage the backs of my hands at least thirty times with each of the three steps of METAMASSAGE. After this initial application, remove the cream with the white towel, carefully shifting it each time you wipe some off. You will be surprised at the dirt you'll see, even though you first washed your hands with soap and water.

Eye Make-up Removal

Remove all eye make-up with remover pads. As you become more expert, you'll be able to remove your eye make-up with cleansing cream and without getting it in your eyes. Be sure not to use tissues around your eyes. Lint is extremely irritating and can cause redness. The wood fibers from the tissues can also penetrate this delicate skin.

THE ROUTINE

The METAMASSAGE routine is composed of three steps. The first time you carry out the procedure, begin by massaging with your cleansing cream 25 to 30 times on each part (figures 1–11) of the face and neck. By liquefying the cream to this count you are removing surface dirt and, if you use it, make-up. You must remove the cream from both face and hands before continuing on to the second step. This procedure is described following the METAMASSAGE technique (p. 58).

The second application of cleansing cream is to soften the epidermis, or top layer of skin, which is chiefly dryness and dead cells. The count increases to 50 times for *each part* of the face and neck. Again, carefully remove all the cream.

The third massage is for softening and smoothing. It must be done 100 times on *each area* of the face and neck. Do not massage the same cleansing cream *into* the skin, but continually add more cream to the face and neck as needed in order to keep your movements fluid.

The Technique

Let your fingers flow smoothly over your skin like a skater glides on ice. Feather touches are what is needed. *Always use enough cleansing cream so that you do not pull the skin.* Apply more if you need to. Pay particular attention to massaging the skin, not the bone. Remember the heat generated from your palm when it was held two inches from your face. Count all the time. The counting is most important and should be followed assiduously; it helps you to concentrate and relax while META-MASSAGING. I recommend that you read through the instructions completely before beginning your META-MASSAGE treatment for the first time.

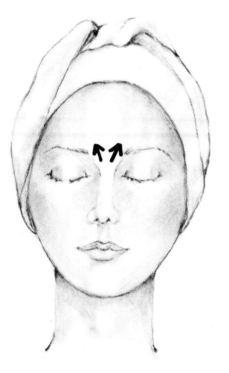

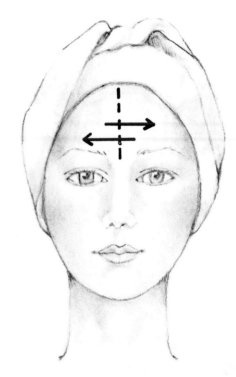

Figure 1 Begin with the area between the eyes, since this is often the center of tension. Massage here in a V-shaped motion, alternately stroking upward on each side, using the middle or ring finger of each hand. Discover which finger is more comfortable and flexible in movement. After stroking upward on one side do not push down (*never* push down on your skin!), but lift your finger, making room to stroke upward on the other side with the other hand. Repeat these upward strokes until you've finished the count.

Figure 2 Picture a line connecting the nose to the hairline and cutting the forehead in half vertically. Using two fingers of each hand, begin at the top (hairline) in the middle of the forehead at the imaginary line and stroke straight across to the side of the head. Work down to the eyebrows, always returning to the center of the forehead to begin each stroke across. Now work back up again, covering the entire forehead area. Alternate using both hands.

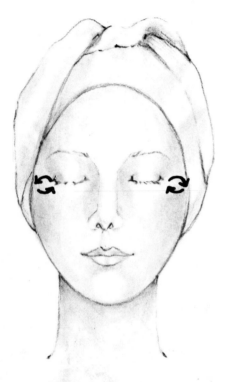

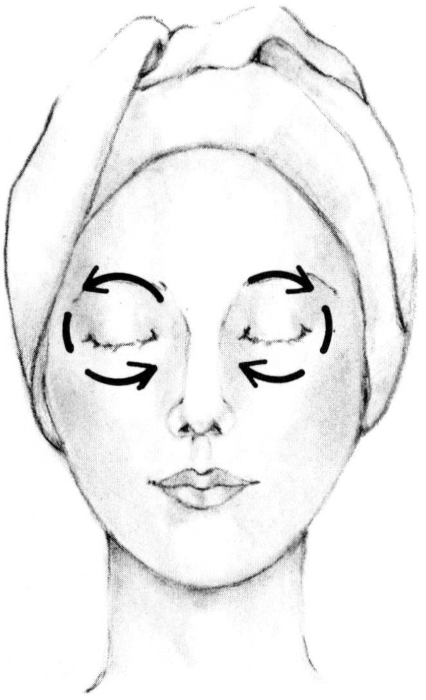

Figure 3 Use both hands *simultaneously*. Again, choose the most comfortable fingers. Make little circular movements on the temples only. Don't move onto the eye socket area... this comes next.

Figure 4 Use the one or two fingers of both hands *simultaneously*. Start on the inner bone of the eyebrow at the bridge of the nose. Make circular motions around the eye socket, across the cheek bone to the inner corner of the eye. Always work gently over the bones. Finish back where you started, making complete circles. The strokes must be continuous and *feather light*. Be careful not to pull the skin directly under the eyes. The skin is very delicate here, as there are no oil glands, and this is generally the first place to show lines.

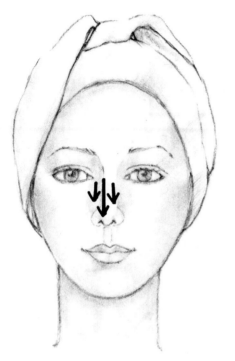 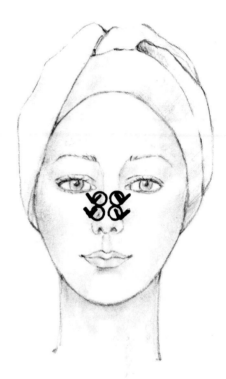

Figures 5 and 6 Work from the bridge of the nose to the tip with straight, downward, alternate strokes, being sure to cover the sides also. You may also alternate these strokes with small, circular, outward motions. Use only the middle or index fingers. Careful cleansing will help eliminate blackheads, a common skin problem in this area.

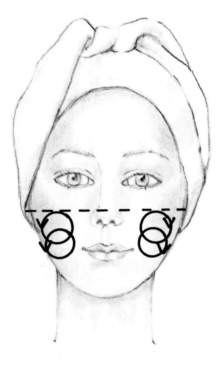 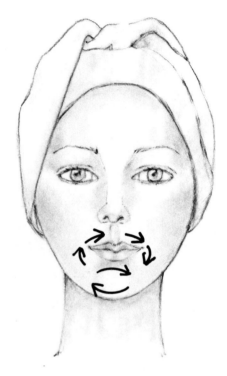

Figure 7 Start below the cheekbone, avoiding the eye area. Make silver-dollar-sized outward motions. Using both hands simultaneously work from the cheekbones to the lower jaw, taking extreme care not to miss any of this extensive portion of the face. Do not go into the mouth and chin area. Two or three fingers can be used. These circles must extend no higher than the middle of the ear opening, avoiding the delicate eye area. Keep your circles uniform in size. If your cheeks move up and down while massaging, you're pressing too hard.

Figure 8 The circular movements around the mouth and chin should overlap to include the lower jaw. With one hand use the third, ring and little finger, working either right to left or left to right.

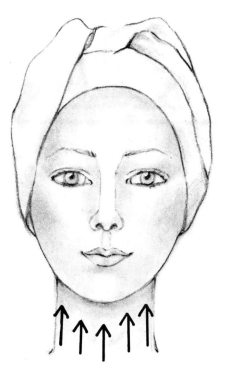 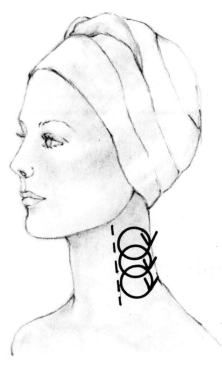

Figures 9 and 10 Use flat fingers of both hands. Alternate strokes upward in absolutely parallel lines from the collarbone to the jaw. If you find parallel lines difficult on the sides of the neck, you may switch to circular outward motions here. Confine the motions only to the area from the back of the ear to the collarbone.

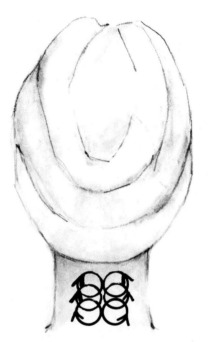

Figure 11 Using three or four fingers, make inward silver-dollar-sized circular motions going from the nape down to the base of the neck and back up again. Use the right hand for the left side of the neck and vice versa.

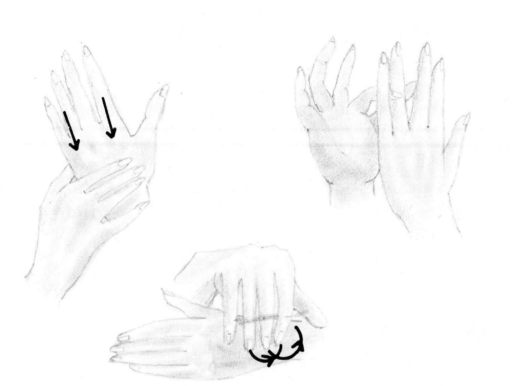

Figure 12 Hands are one of the first parts of the body to look old. For this reason, be sure to massage your hands after each of the three METAMASSAGE steps. This will reduce loss of elasticity through better circulation, replace moisture lost naturally through dehydration and have the same smoothing effect as you'll see in your face and neck. Rub the backs of your hands, paying particular attention to the wrists. Count twenty-five circular motions on the top side of each wrist. It is amazing to see how these epidermal bracelets can be smoothed out.

Don't neglect the fingers, either. Start from the tips and go all the way down each one several times in a snake-like movement.

Motions for treatment of the hands should always start from the fingers, working down along the back of the hand just over the wrist. Never push the other way from the wrist down; this is thin and delicate skin.

Proper treatment of the hands is most important. Plastic surgery can't help you here.

Removal of the Cream

The cream must be removed *after each of the three applications*, and don't forget the hands, wrists and under the nails each time as well. Please remember that each area has its designated movement and is unique unto itself. Review each one carefully before beginning the procedure so that you can begin with confidence.

Forehead

The "V" area will be taken care of when you remove the cream from the forehead. Place the towel just over the center line (Figure 2), and gently, but firmly, slide the towel across the forehead to the hairline. Working your way along the towel to a clean portion, do exactly the same thing on the other side.

Temples and Eyes

The temples do not require a circular motion for cream removal. Feather-whisk along the hairline only. When removing the cream in a circular motion around the eyes, the temple will be taken care of in the process. Be careful not to pull on the delicate eye tissue. Work on the bone in the eye socket area. It is not necessary to rub the eyelids. Gently blot without pulling the skin.

Nose

Use a downward motion from the bridge of the nose along the sides ending with the creases at the nostril. Also make a downward motion from the bridge on top of the nose to the tip.

Cheeks, Jawline and Chin

Cover the palm and back of the hand with the towel. With the index finger, begin midway at the nose. Place palm flat on the cheek and use a sliding motion rolling onto the little finger as you go straight across to the middle of the ear opening. Use the same motion on the left side, this time covering the palm as before; but, beginning with the little finger midway at the nose, roll the palm in a straight line to the middle of the ear opening. For the jawline, begin in the middle of the chin and with an upward motion move along the bone only...being careful always not to stretch the skin.

Mouth

Use a circular motion around the mouth, paying special attention to the corners of the lips.

Neck

Using the same motion as when you put on the cream, remove it with the same parallel lines and the flat portion of the palm. This applies to the front and the sides. The back of the neck is a downward motion from the hairline to the base of the column to the collarbone.

Hands

Be as meticulous about removing the cream from your hands as you have been with your face and neck. Remember to use the towel under the nails after each treatment. Spend a lit-

each eye with pads in the prescribed direction. Always move to a new space on the cotton as you did on the towel. Pull the cotton apart, using it back to back. Try not to frown or raise the eyebrows while doing this. You may close your eyes, but do not bear down on the upper eyelids. Gently blot this delicate area.

Use of Astringent

Now saturate (but not sloppy wet) more cotton pads with astringent. Start with the forehead and go over the rest of the face and neck as you did when removing the cream. Carefully avoid the eye area. There are no oil glands here and astringent would be unnecessarily drying. Whisk upward along the hairline to remove any excess cream.

tle extra time around the cuticles to soften them. Whisk, using a cotton pad moistened with astringent, after the cream removal and then apply your moisturizer. Apply a tad extra in circular motions on those epidermal bracelet lines. Again, don't neglect the fingers. Cleanse them, using the same snake-like movement as when you treated them. The feeling is so soothing you won't want to quit.

Hygienic Precaution

Hands carry more microbes than the mouth. It is safer to kiss than to shake hands. Do not let anyone dip into your cream or use your white towel. You must move your white towel to a clean portion each time you remove the cream from any area of the face, neck and hands.

Start at the end of the towel on one side and work along it horizontally. There is no sense taking cream off one side of the forehead, for instance, and rubbing that same cream onto the other side. Be conservative in your use of space, and be meticulous overall. You will get used to it. You will also be amazed at the grime and dead cell debris that appear on your white towel.

POST METAMASSAGE

Removal of Excess Cream

Touch your face and neck gently in each area. If you feel you have not removed all the cream, feather-whisk each place gently to clean any residue, using the motions described for that area. After the three repetitions of cleansing and removal, check in a mirror for excess cream as you perform the last steps. Pay particular attention to the hairline and always check behind the earlobes for cream you might have missed.

Bathing of Eyes

Take two cotton pads or a sizable piece of cotton wool. Dip in cold water, gently squeezing out the excess. Go around

—And Moisturizer

Since the METAMASSAGE technique works to balance your skin, you will only need a small amount of moisturizer around the eyes and on the full neck column. If you METAMASSAGE regularly, any more than that will prove excessive and can result in clogged pores. Pat the moisturizer around the eye area (with the now well-learned motions) until it is absorbed. Gently rub in the moisturizer as you go up the front of the neck. On the side and back use the inward, circular motions. Do not go below the collarbone. Treat only the areas your METAMASSAGE has cleansed.

A Final Touch

Take your magnifying mirror again and carefully examine your skin texture and pores. Notice the glow and relaxed countenance your soothing procedure has accomplished. Your skin is clean, fresh and free of tension. From the first time you METAMASSAGE you will see surprising results.

For an added touch, take an old, clean toothbrush or eyebrow brush and use it to brush your eyebrows upward, then straight across. This trains them to lie smoothly.

Should Break Out Occur

Once you begin to METAMASSAGE daily and your skin balances itself, many of the blemishes underneath the outer layer of the skin will surface as you cleanse and soften the epidermis. Don't be alarmed if in the first two weeks you appear to break out. This is exactly what you want. Your cells are renewing themselves continually. By clearing the dead layer you are allowing the new, healthy cells to mature and thrive. You are assisting a complex chemical process that nourishes and supplies energy through increased circulation and unimpeded cell replacement. METAMASSAGE creates healthy skin which expands to its naturally firm shape and gives immediate results from the first time you do it!

Constantly remind yourself not to *squint, frown or stretch* your skin by resting your hands on your face. Also, I know how tempting it is to put your hand on an undercover bump, or on the surfaced pimple. In the first case this can irritate. In the latter case it can cause infection by transmission of bacteria.

If a pimple should surface before you go to bed put a small dab of dry cornstarch, mask (one of the commercial kind that dries) or white iodine (if it does not irritate your skin) on it, especially just as the sore begins to emerge. This technique is particularly helpful during the first two weeks of METAMASSAGE. You'll be helping those annoying, below-the-skin blemishes to surface and dry.

The Morning After

The recommended routine the morning after METAMASSAGING is to wash your face with whatever soap you usually use. If you have sensitive skin or an allergy and cannot use soap then splash your face and neck with tepid water several times. Be sure to cover all areas, including the hairline.

There are so many non-allergic soaps now available that surely you can find one that suits your skin. Some people find great success with "Noxema," "Neutrogena," "Johnson's Baby Soap" or one of the liquid non-soap scrubs made by Germaine Monteil, 2nd Debut or any reputable cosmetic house. These products are effective and non-drying.

Dry the face and neck with the usual whisk-touch motions according to figures 1–11 and pat dry any excess moisture.

Apply moisturizer around the eyes, neck and on the hands. You can use a different, less heavy one than what you used the night before. Apply make-up if you wish or leave your skin free of any encumbrances (unless you wish to pat on dry cornstarch, avoiding the area around the eyes) for the day. Either way, you'll glow!

Note: You can leave the cornstarch on as long as you wish. With a *"Co-et"* cotton pad or a clean powder puff, different from the powder puff you use for powder, gently whisk off the surplus that has not naturally fallen off.

Cleansing grains are a good idea

tle extra time around the cuticles to soften them. Whisk, using a cotton pad moistened with astringent, after the cream removal and then apply your moisturizer. Apply a tad extra in circular motions on those epidermal bracelet lines. Again, don't neglect the fingers. Cleanse them, using the same snake-like movement as when you treated them. The feeling is so soothing you won't want to quit.

Hygienic Precaution

Hands carry more microbes than the mouth. It is safer to kiss than to shake hands. Do not let anyone dip into your cream or use your white towel. You must move your white towel to a clean portion each time you remove the cream from any area of the face, neck and hands.

Start at the end of the towel on one side and work along it horizontally. There is no sense taking cream off one side of the forehead, for instance, and rubbing that same cream onto the other side. Be conservative in your use of space, and be meticulous overall. You will get used to it. You will also be amazed at the grime and dead cell debris that appear on your white towel.

POST METAMASSAGE

Removal of Excess Cream

Touch your face and neck gently in each area. If you feel you have not removed all the cream, feather-whisk each place gently to clean any residue, using the motions described for that area. After the three repetitions of cleansing and removal, check in a mirror for excess cream as you perform the last steps. Pay particular attention to the hairline and always check behind the earlobes for cream you might have missed.

Bathing of Eyes

Take two cotton pads or a sizable piece of cotton wool. Dip in cold water, gently squeezing out the excess. Go around each eye with pads in the prescribed direction. Always move to a new space on the cotton as you did on the towel. Pull the cotton apart, using it back to back. Try not to frown or raise the eyebrows while doing this. You may close your eyes, but do not bear down on the upper eyelids. Gently blot this delicate area.

Use of Astringent

Now saturate (but not sloppy wet) more cotton pads with astringent. Start with the forehead and go over the rest of the face and neck as you did when removing the cream. Carefully avoid the eye area. There are no oil glands here and astringent would be unnecessarily drying. Whisk upward along the hairline to remove any excess cream.

twice a week, or even three times for excessively oily skins. After META-MASSAGING for a while you'll find your skin overall will normalize, then you'll only need the cleansing grains once a week. You can also use corn meal or rolled oats instead of commercial cleansing grains. Merely make a paste with water and roll gently in circular motions over your face and neck. After rinsing thoroughly, pat your skin dry, don't rub. Put moisturizer on the neck and around the eyes only. As you will see in the section on Masks (p. 81), many of the products used are things you have at home.

You'll want to keep a box of cornstarch handy, especially during the first two weeks of your treatments. After you've completed the METAMASSAGE procedure (including moisturizing), use the cornstarch every night before you go to bed. With a *Co-et* or clean powder puff, gently pat the dry cornstarch over every portion of the face and under the jawline if there are any skin eruptions, with the exception of the eye area. Leave it on all night or, if someone is going to accuse you of rushing Halloween, whisk it off after ten minutes. The cornstarch will absorb any excess cream you might have missed during the first two-week learning process. If you METAMASSAGE before going out in the evening or in the morning, leave the cornstarch on for five minutes, then lightly brush it off, being careful to remove it all. Apply your make-up as usual.

A Check List

Have you memorized the motions for each part of the face and neck?

Are you remembering to do the top part of the wrists and hands and cuticles?

Do you go under the nails with the towel each time you remove the cream?

Are you using clean, white towels?

Are you moving the towel when taking off the cream?

Are you using enough cream so as not to pull the skin?

Do you use water around the eyes?

Are you remembering to whisk around the hairline and clean behind the ears when using the astringent?

Are you putting moisturizer only around the eye area, the neck and hands?

Are you honestly counting 25, 50 and 100 times on each area during the three separate applications of the cleansing cream?

Are you removing the cream after each
application?

Important Note: Avoid being aggressive in
your massaging, as this will stretch the
skin! Remember to use a light, feathery
touch.

IF YOU HAVE HAD COSMETIC SURGERY

Post-Operative Care

For those of you who have had face lifts and eye lifts, METAMASSAGE is invaluable. You will preserve your firm, new skin without having to think of surgery again. Follow the instructions as given, paying special attention to smoothing the skin, not tugging at it. Get to know your bone structure so that you can work gently over the skin on these solid foundations.

To minimize incision lines after your full METAMASSAGE, apply Vitamin E or castor oil to these areas for a full month or longer. You may start your full METAMASSAGE treatment as soon as the soreness is lessened, but check with your doctor if you have any hesitation.

Post-Operative Maintenance

During your recuperative period METAMASSAGE both morning and evening before bed. The increased circulation will hasten the healing process. I suggest this dual treatment for at least two weeks. You may then return to the usual morning after routine, only METAMASSAGING at night. Do, however, remember to use moisturizer around the eyes and on the full neck column.

Cornstarch

What was good for baby rashes fifty years ago is excellent for inflammation and redness after plastic surgery today. Following the METAMASSAGE and post-treatment (astringent-moisturizer) gently pat dry cornstarch on your face with a cotton pad. Avoid the eye area. Leave it on all night and it will disappear by itself. Repeat the application any time you wish. You may want to apply the cornstarch for fifteen minutes before you go out. Do so and whisk away the excess with a soft complexion brush, cotton pad or powder puff before applying make-up. It is one of the best skin equalizers available.

METAMASSAGE is perfect for maintaining your present good fortune. Put some discipline into your life and you'll prevent the necessity of future surgery. Constantly remind yourself not to squint, frown or use exaggerated facial expressions. Let your eyes, voice and body language speak. Refrain from putting your hands on your face. Leaning or propping your face on them can stretch the skin. Become acquainted with the feeling of frowning and squinting. When you feel that you are doing so, gently touch that area and consciously relax the muscles.

Your decision to have a face lift was monumental. Relax, be aware and start anew in your skin care routine. And, most important, *enjoy* it!

SUNBATHING AND METAMASSAGE

We have all heard often enough how detrimental too much sun is for the skin. Yet there are beneficial effects to sunbathing if we do not diminish them by abuse. I never sit in the sun without having METAMASSAGED either the night before or just before sunbathing if, for some reason, I was unable to do my routine before retiring. I also prefer to bathe before sunning. If I am only going to lie out thirty minutes to an hour, the moisturizing body lotion I use after the bath is sufficient for protection from burning. If I know I'll be exposed to the sun for a much longer period of time, I substitute a tanning balm for body lotion, and a sun screen where experience has taught me it is necessary. You may find that more protection is needed, depending on your skin type. Softening and cleansing the skin before sunning, however, tends to give a more even tan and prevents drying. Remember that soap and water can diminish the beneficial effects of the ultraviolet rays of the sun, so I always wait at least two hours *after* sunning if I feel it necessary to bathe again. Try it; you'll be pleasantly surprised at how beautifully and evenly you tan. And your skin feels soft and wonderful!

SLEEPING AND SKIN CARE

A French doctor, Gustav Mathieu, did extensive research on insomnia and concluded the following: if your head is pointing *north* you sleep more soundly; *east*, you sleep uneasily; *west*, you might have high blood pressure and *south*, you could have indigestion. Try experimenting on your own and see if his findings are helpful to you.

Sleeping position is also important. There are many schools of thought on this subject. The position most agree is the best is one of lying on the back with one leg bent at a forty-five-degree angle. This position creates greater lung capacity so breathing is not impaired, and the one bent leg relieves strain on the pelvic area. Ideally the arms shouldn't be parallel to the body but at right angles to the shoulders with the forearms straight up, palms up and open.

Certainly for the benefit of the skin, the on-the-back position is the preferred one. Along with the impaired breathing capacity, pressure on various organs and tensed muscles in the facial and neck areas, certain sleeping positions in which the skin is contorted or stretched can create severe wrinkles.

If you are accustomed to sleeping with a pillow, try to break the habit. Doctors, however, often recommend a pillow for certain respiratory difficulties. Whether or not this recommendation applies to you, if you *must* use a pillow, be sure your skin is smoothed and your face is flat when you sleep on your stomach or favorite side. By becoming aware of your sleeping position and the harm it can do to your skin, you'll learn to change your slumber habits.

We make approximately 140 movements during eight hours of sleep. Sleep is not cessation of activity, but rather a different form of behavior. Begin to notice the structure of people's faces—you can observe which side of the face they usually sleep on from the long, vertical lines on their forehead or cheeks. Try sleeping on your back without a pillow, as pillows restrict circulation in the neck in addition to creasing the skin.

Do not wear restrictive clothing when you sleep. Be comfortable! I don't know what percentage of the population sleeps in the nude but if it suits you, do it. Your body temperature will tell you if you get too warm or too cold at night. Open windows, air conditioners or electric blankets are a matter of taste and locale. Don't be afraid to try different articles of dress or undress or various room temperatures. The important thing is that you sleep well. Sleep is the time your body requires and uses to repair itself.

There are psychological threads and strains of the physiological weaving through the individual patterns of sleep. To calm your mind and relax yourself I *do* suggest beginning your repose at any hour, even when napping, with the following exercise:

Lie down flat on your back, legs straight, feet relaxed, arms parallel to the body, palms up. Exhale through the mouth, then breathe in gently though the nose and, with your natural rhythm, exhale smoothly while consciously telling your whole body to relax. Beginning with the toes, work up through each part of the body, commanding each area to relax individually. When you have relaxed your entire body begin again, working downward from the neck to the face.

Remember, there are voluntary and involuntary muscles in the face which reflect your thoughts and feelings. Each time you instruct those facial muscles to relax, you will sense a definite lessening of tension. Sleep well. As William Shakespeare said, "Our foster nurse of nature is repose." After your META-MASSAGE you will find you definitely sleep better and will awaken refreshed, even with few hours of sleep.

......
MASKS

Masks not only feel wonderful but they also have a soothing effect. They minimize large pores, help to remove dead cells from the epidermis and increase the circulation. Use them three times a week the first month of your META-MASSAGE program if you have oily

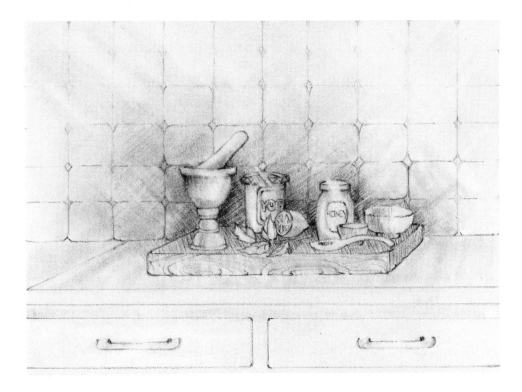

skin, and once a week if your skin is dry. Once your skin is normalized you may use them as little (once a week) or as often as you like. They are a great pick-me-up any time. Try one before a party or festive occasion for that special glow.

There are herbal masks, masks that dry and are washed off with tepid water or cold water and masks that peel off. Whatever suits you is what's important, whether it's made from ingredients in your own kitchen or bought at a cosmetic counter. There are so many choices these days that shopping around should be fun. I don't believe some are better for dry or oily skin, because with METAMASSAGE your skin becomes normalized. You can use just about any mask as long as it is not irritating to your skin. It's nice to have two or three different kinds. Some are good for a quick pick-me-up while others require a longer time. For those that require more time to set, cover your face (except for the eye socket area) and neck area. Try not to talk for fifteen minutes.

Take the opportunity to lie on a flat surface with your feet raised about 18 inches (or whatever is comfortable) higher than your level body. If you have a slant board use it. Follow the

Mask Recipes

Add to	sour cream mayonnaise or yogurt	unflavored gelatin egg white	Rhine wine champagne or vodka
		any of the following:	
For oily skin	pineapple papaya castor oil avocado honey	salt sugar banana celery leaves watermelon	lemon juice strawberry mashed grape cinnamon oil
for dry skin	castor oil avocado honey strawberry banana celery leaves	salt watermelon sugar pear	cucumber cinnamon oil corn meal
Slice in	petals of rose, marigold or bachelor button		
Sprinkle in	mint, rosemary, parsley and camomile		

relaxation technique described on p. 79

The ideal method of mixing the ingredients for your mask recipes is with a blender. You will need one-half to one cup of mask mixture, depending on which ingredients you choose and the thickness you prefer. If you do not have a blender then a mortar and pestle or a potato masher will work to combine your ingredients. Don't be afraid to experiment!

After you've applied the mask and are in a reclining position, start with the hair, scalp and facial muscles and do the relaxation exercises working *down* over each part of the body and then back up again. You'll look and feel relaxed and peaceful.

Afterward, remove the mask using tepid to cool water, pat dry, and use moisturizer around the eyes and the underneath chin and neck areas. Don't use quick-dry masks on the neck until you have normalized your skin with METAMASSAGE.

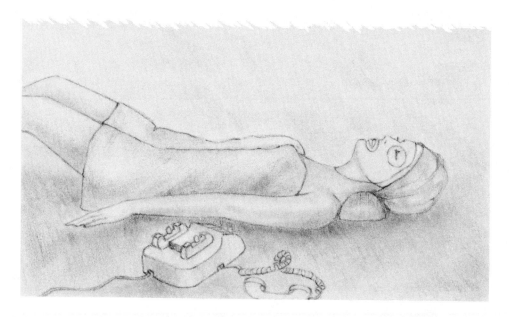

Gently rub on after the mask, for that extra feeling of freshness: sliced potato, cucumber, papaya, apricot, honey dew, aloe vera, lemon or cantaloupe.

As a variation, try using wet but squeezed-out tea bags over the eyes or even sliced cucumbers. A trick my mother used to use was to moisten cotton pads with a diluted mixture of witch hazel and distilled water and refrigerate them a few minutes before applying. This is a particularly good feeling because of the coolness of the eye pads, and helps to alleviate swelling around the eyes.

Try some of the various combinations given here and do enjoy. Masks are a luxury.

YOUR HAIR

Have you ever noticed that your hair seems to have a personality all its own? How often must you do battle with your hair? Stubbornly resistant to your wish, independent of your will, hair carries on with its idiosyncrasies and usually wins. Cowlicks, swirls, waves—curly or straight, thin or fat hair—all are formidable opponents. They can, however, be subdued by a few well-chosen counter-offensives.

Your diet plays an important part in the quality of your hair. Good scalp circulation increases strength and growth. Thorough washing, rinsing and conditioning all contribute to beautiful hair. Brushing, combing and arranging your hair are equally important when done properly. As we must take care of our health from within, we must also improve ourselves from without. Well-cared-for hair will provide a suitable frame for a beautiful complexion.

Brushing and Combing

The top layers of hair are not as strong as the crescent moon area from ear to ear around the base of the skull. Bending over and brushing hair forward from the back of the head helps the texture and sheen of your hair, and protects the weaker top strands. Try it.

Bend over and begin by brushing forward from the base of the skull to

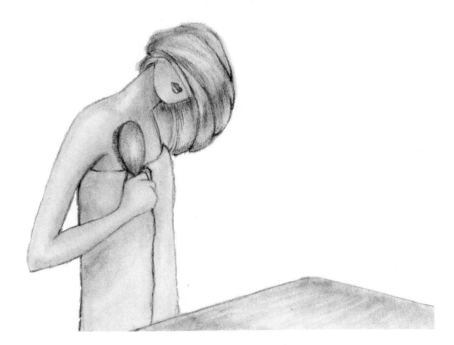

the top of the crown of the head. Then, starting at the right temple, brush just over the crown overlapping to the left side and vice versa. Be careful not to pull as you continue your strokes down the hair shafts to the ends. Thirty to fifty strokes at a time are sufficient. You are extending your massage method to an appendage of the skin, that is, the hair. Treat it with the same consideration as you do the rest of your body. Brushing and combing the top layers are useful for arranging the hair, but the basic premise of hair treatment—brushing from the base of the skull—is to stimulate the blood vessels below the bulb of each hair shaft.

Washing Technique

We are fortunate to have many wonderful and pure shampoos to choose from. Experiment but try to find one prepared with pure fats and oils and with as few chemicals as possible. If you have a scalp condition this is a different problem that may require medical attention.

Wet your hair and pour some shampoo in the palm of your hand, lique-fying it by rubbing between the palms. Begin to rub gently over the top layers of the hair, working your way to the scalp. With the pads of your fingers, not the nails, massage the upper periphery of the scalp from the hairline, over the crown and temples to the base of the skull. With your thumbs begin in the middle of the lower cranium and with circular motions massage outward to the ears and back again. With the palms of both hands, simultaneously brush over the top layers of the hair, continuing to the ends of the strands.

Rinse well with water, never too hot or too cold. Now you may either use a prepared conditioner or a creation of your own. The squeak test really works once you've gotten all the soap out of your hair!

Wash your hair as often as is necessary, depending on your particular body chemistry, where you live, the amount of dust and pollution in the air and your physical activities. For some people washing once a week is adequate. For others every day is not too often. You be the judge of the frequency you need to shampoo.

Rinses

A rinse both conditions and highlights the hair. There are many excellent products on the market, but it is fun to prepare your own. Natural products found in your pantry or spice cabinet are not only pure and readily available, but are economical as well. Try experimenting with some of the following:

- —Orange or Rose Water mixed half and half with a pint of water is like an aphrodisiac, and should be used as often as possible. The glorious smell is the turn-on!
- —For redheads and brunettes, one teaspoon of apple cider vinegar to each pint of water not only balances the pH factor, but softens the hair.
- —Three teaspoons of cinnamon steeped in one pint of warm water are aromatic and highlight brown hair.
- —For blondes, one-half freshly squeezed lemon in a pint of water gives sheen and body to the hair.
- —Four teaspoons or six tea bags of comfrey in one quart of water regenerate aging tissues and are an effective cell proliferant.

Pour the rinse on the hair, leave on for at least one minute then rinse the hair with clean, tepid water.

Alternative Treatments for the Hair and Scalp

The following suggestions are treatments for the hair and scalp that were used before many of the products on the market were conceived. You might ask your mother or grandmother what they used to treat their hair. Natural products are still preferable to chemically compounded commercial ones.

- —Rosemary leaves steeped in hot water which are then used to wet the hair completely one hour before washing will brighten dull hair. After you've steeped the leaves wrapped in a piece of cheesecloth, squeeze out the excess liquid and rub the leaves onto the scalp. Rinse the hair with the water used to steep the leaves and wrap hair with a towel before washing it an hour later. This is particularly good for brown or black hair.
- —For light hair, do as the Romans used

to do. Follow the above instructions but steep camomile instead of rosemary leaves and apply to the hair.

Save the water in which you cook artichokes and massage your scalp with it if you have dandruff.

Oil Wrap

A simple old world remedy for dull, listless hair is the Oil Wrap. My Lebanese ancestors used olive oil. My contemporaries use olive oil, avocado oil, almond oil, oil of apricots, or safflower or castor oil. I prefer the olive or castor oil. One usually has a bottle around the house, and the quicker it is used the better. Eating rancid oil or applying it externally can rob the body of vitamin A.

There is no mystery to application of the oil; it does not even have to be heated. Heat is not good for the hair; and this includes too hot water, too vigorous brushing, hair dryers and the sun. Like prepared sake or bath water, your body heat is the most healthful temperature for you.

Rub the oil between your palms to warm and even the consistency. According to the length of the hair, grasp it at the nape of the neck, sliding both hands down the length of the strands to the ends. Then rub the ends between your palms. Part the hair into three sections and with the same motions, but with alternating hands, be sure you cover every strand.

Rub more oil between your palms and from the hairline over the crown lightly smooth over the top portion of the hair. Do not get oil on the scalp. Food for the scalp comes from the bloodstream. Oil can congest the sweat pores. To treat the scalp use a gentle fingertip massage, or brush as described in the "Brushing and Combing" section.

If you wish, a moist, warm towel can be used for a wet wrap or aluminum foil for a dry one. Cover the entire head for two to four hours with either one of these wraps. Depending on your time schedule, leave it on as long as possible. Then wash and set or dry your hair as usual.

As an alternate shorter wrap you may use mashed avocados, mayonnaise or yogurt. Lanolin is a bit heavy but if it's used sparingly and liquefied it becomes very effective. Again, any pure fats or oils will do. Leave on from fifteen minutes until what your time schedule will allow, following up with your usual wash and set or blow drying. But watch that heat! It can dry out your hair.

Egg Prep

Eggs are abundant in protein and amino acids. Keratin, a form of protein found in eggs, is the main component of hair and nails. Egg conditions the hair and gives it body. The Egg Prep is particularly effective after the Oil Wrap, which should be applied without rinsing or washing your hair first.

To prepare your Egg Prep, beat both the white and yolk of one egg until there is no separation. Apply the blend to the whole head, covering every strand. Gently rub the egg into the hair as if you were shampooing. When you are through the egg should not drip. If it does, continue the shampooing motion. For long hair be sure you work the egg down to the ends, then attach the hair with a clip to the top of the head. Do the Egg Prep fifteen minutes before your bath or shower, allowing time for it to dry while you bathe. Leave on thirty minutes if you can. Let the egg dry naturally and do not wrap as the egg will become thin and runny.

Be sure to use the Egg Prep *after* the Oil Wrap for optimum body and sheen. The egg will also start to absorb some of the oil from your hair and give it body.

For an overnight heat treatment, put the oil on two-thirds of the length of your hair (to avoid clogging the scalp) and cover your head with a plastic bag.

For short hair, rub the oil between the fingers and gently grasp the hair an inch above the roots, continually applying the oil to the ends of the strands. Place more oil between the palms, rub the palms together lightly and smooth over the entire top layer of the scalp from upper hairline to lower hairline.

Be sure, after this intensive treatment, to wash, using two separate latherings, and experiment with one of the suggested rinses in the RINSE section.

After the oil treatment, if you do not use the Egg Prep, apply shampoo to the hair *before* wetting it when you wash. Leave on for five or ten minutes, then wet the hair and lather well. Rinse thoroughly, lather again and massage the scalp with the pads of your fingers, not the nails. Rinse well with warm, then cool water to increase circulation.

Justice Hair Pack

A friend of mine, Jeff Justice of *Clark Savon Hair Studio* in Los Angeles, California, is an expert on hair who swears by this secret formula for a hair pack. He says it is the best he has used in thirty years of hair dressing. I am delighted to be able to pass it on to you. The Justice Pack helps relieve over-porous hair that has been aggravated by too much bleaching, dyeing or permanent waving. Poor texture, limpness and broken or split ends due to abuse of the hair or too much sun will be alleviated by using the pack once or twice a week. For normal hair once every two weeks is sufficient. You may use the pack one week after a permanent wave on normal hair. If after a permanent the hair is frizzy, then use the pack after seventy-two hours. Wrapping the head during the pack is not necessary with this fantastic conditioner.

Measure equal parts, one-half cup each, of Jojoba Oil and Aloe Vera Gel. Add 4,000 I.U. (International Units), or 4 capsules of 1,000 I.U. each, of vitamin E and one capsule of vitamin A containing 10,000 I.U. These ingredients can be found in any health food store. Cut off the ends of the capsules with a small pair of scissors. Mix everything together with an egg in a blender. Apply to the hair, work it in thoroughly and leave on for one hour. Wash, blow dry or set the hair as usual and see what Justice is done!

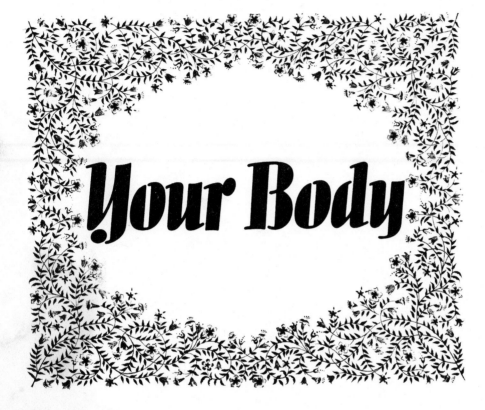

Your Body

INTRODUCTION TO BODY RITUAL AND ROUTINE

From the time of birth we are unalterably aging. Whether you are aware of it or not, a person's age affects your attitude toward them. But life is an infinitely more interesting tapestry when you can defy the normal concepts of age and aging. Psychological, social, moral and anatomical age exist at different levels in any one person. Chronological age need not dictate our entire personality, or attitude about ourselves.

Dr. Elisabeth Kübler-Ross says, "It is fear and guilt that are the only enemies of man, and if we have the courage to face our own fears and guilts and unfinished business, we will emerge more self-respecting and self-loving and more courageous to face whatever windstorms come in our direction."

Ritual is a great part of life. We have ceremonies for marriage, birthdays and numerous special events. How you care for yourself and maintain your body is also a ritual. Good grooming and physical fitness require habits that must be repeated over and over again for lasting results. Every night before going to bed, one undresses, removes make-up, hopefully METAMASSAGES, perhaps takes a bath/shower, brushes teeth and hair, then redresses (unless you buff it). In the morning or before dressing for some social event is another ritual of habits. The point is to make the most of your efforts in whatever time you allow yourself.

METAMASSAGE is a compilation of Energy Replacement exercises which will not only aid your body externally but help it to function efficiently. With tender loving care you can realize your full potential now.

The METAMASSAGE *Bathing Routine* is based on the same theory as the facial massage. By aiding circulation and removing superfluous dead cells from the epidermis, you retard the aging process. Toned muscles prevent loss of elasticity in the skin and replacement of moisture prevents dehydration.

You will make the best use of your time and in fact conserve time and energy by disciplining yourself in this method of skin care. Like the facial massage, the very first application of the METAMASSAGE bathing principles will make you feel and look different. Bathing becomes a great experience rather than just a necessity. It is a large part of my survival technique. Aside from its physical benefits, this ritual helps me to maintain self-confidence and a sense of well-being and increases my energy level.

Having roughed it in Third World countries for many years, I find nothing as satisfactory as my own tub, bathing essentials and plenty of hot water for relaxation and refreshment. Adapt I have, however, and in the midst of a wilderness I seek a pond, lake or some form of water to scrub and wash. I find I can't think as well if this water therapy isn't available. One of the prime points in the *Armed Forces Manual* on survival technique is to seek water—naturally for drinking purposes—and just as important, for bathing the body every day. Cleanliness of body increases sharpness of mind. Awareness is part of survival, too.

The METAMASSAGE *Bathing Technique*, from beginning to end, including the cream massage, should take only twenty minutes. There is no scarcity of time, only of initiative.

......

MUSCLES, NERVES AND GLANDS

There are over five hundred muscles in the human body which comprise approximately half of its weight. The three classifications of muscles are *voluntary*, *involuntary* and *cardiac*. Your voluntary muscles are controlled by will and are ruled by the cerebro-spinal nervous system. The involuntary muscles function without will, controlled by the sympathetic nervous system. The function of the cardiac muscle, relating to the heart, is evident. Not only do muscles shape the body, there could be no movement without them.

Muscles can be stimulated by the following methods: acids and salts, massage, electric currents, infrared and ultraviolet rays and nerve impulses.

Nerves are long white cords made up of cell processes which carry messages to every part of your body. Stress, muscular fatigue and/or excessive worry are conveyed through the nerves and can deplete your body's store of energy and increase waste products in the system.

Nerves can be stimulated in approximately the same ways as muscles. Proper massage stimulates circulation and is one of the best methods of relieving both muscular and nerve fatigue. Good circulation is vital for health and beauty and necessary for maintaining healthy hair, skin and nails.

The blood and nerves are intimately connected to the glands, which are important in their ability to remove toxins and other elements from the blood. The nervous system controls the functional abilities of the glands.

Massage and wet heat stimulate the muscles, nerves and blood vessels, which in turn assist the glands in breaking up toxins in the bloodstream. This process produces relaxation and lowers the stress and anxiety levels.

AMES BODY ALIGNMENT

Because we rarely breathe correctly, we use less than one-half the normal capacity of our lungs. Therefore, there is not enough exchange of oxygen in the bloodstream to give maximum energy, producing the feelings of lethargy we hear spoken of so often. With optimum energy we accomplish more and as a result feel happier. Skin, hair, nails and, for that matter, all body organs improve with proper breathing as oxygen clears the bloodstream. Breathing is the essence of life. Just as we did the cleansing breath in the mental preparation for METAMASSAGE for the face, let us exchange the old, stale breath for new before the bath/shower.

Totty Ames, a *hatha yoga* teacher in Los Angeles, who started Raquel Welch and Jill St. John, among other luminaries, on their yoga routine, proposes the following exercises to maintain a supple spine and proper posture. When my yoga teacher of twenty-two years died I was not that schooled in the *hatha*, or physical, aspect of yoga.

Only through Miss Ames did I begin to practice the discipline of stretching and breathing, which I religiously carry out every day of my life now.

How your body feels when you first awaken sets the tone for the whole day. You can gain as many benefits from stretching and breathing with concentrated attention as you can out of jogging or calisthenics. In fact, it would be helpful to do these stretching and breathing exercises before *any* strenuous workout. Rarely is attention directed toward your inner self while physically over-exerting your body. One should attempt to create harmony between the mind and body. Without this balance one is wasting time. Physical exercise without self-awareness is merely physical exertion.

To begin these exercises, proper body alignment is extremely important. Any slumping or spinal curvature will constrict the lung capacity. Therefore, concentrate on standing straight and you'll help alleviate many respiratory problems. Your attitude is reflected through posture. Our goal is to place the mind and body in harmony.

The following are four simple series of breathing and body alignment exercises that will enhance your total energy level. Put aside five minutes before your bath or shower to do them.

You may do one, two or all three of the complete breath exercises at one standing, or do five of just one of them if you wish to change your routine. Remind yourself at all times to keep your body straight, your shoulders level and your head erect. *Always* exhale before inhaling as you begin your exercises.

Always breathe in through the nose and exhale through the mouth in these exercises, keeping the lips relaxed. The purpose for breathing in through the nose is to fill the lungs more completely with slower, more deliberate breaths. Exhaling through the mouth accelerates the clearing of wastes in the system, and creates greater lung capacity for fresh air.

Just before performing the *Stretching* or *Hang Loose* exercise take a deep breath and forcibly exhale through the mouth, emptying the lungs before beginning your new breath.

Relax and put your mind at rest. Think of the serene setting you used in mental preparation for METAMASSAGING your face. Try to maintain the picture in your mind as you are doing your *Stretching and Breathing* exercises.

Hang Loose

Stand erect. Place the feet shoulder width apart (or a comfortable distance). Legs tight, knees straight. Arms straight by the sides. Exhale. Breathe deeply in through the nose. Fill lungs to capacity and tighten the whole body. Exhale through the mouth, simultaneously bending forward with the arms coming over the shoulders and touching the floor. If possible place palms flat on the floor, fingertips touching.

Tighten the stomach muscles. Let the head and neck relax. Hold to the count of five. Inhale through the nose and slowly rise to starting position. Repeat five times, stretching farther to the floor with each exhalation. Don't strain. Your spine will become more flexible with constancy and relaxation. For those of you who are very limber the extreme position is with your elbows and hands on the floor.

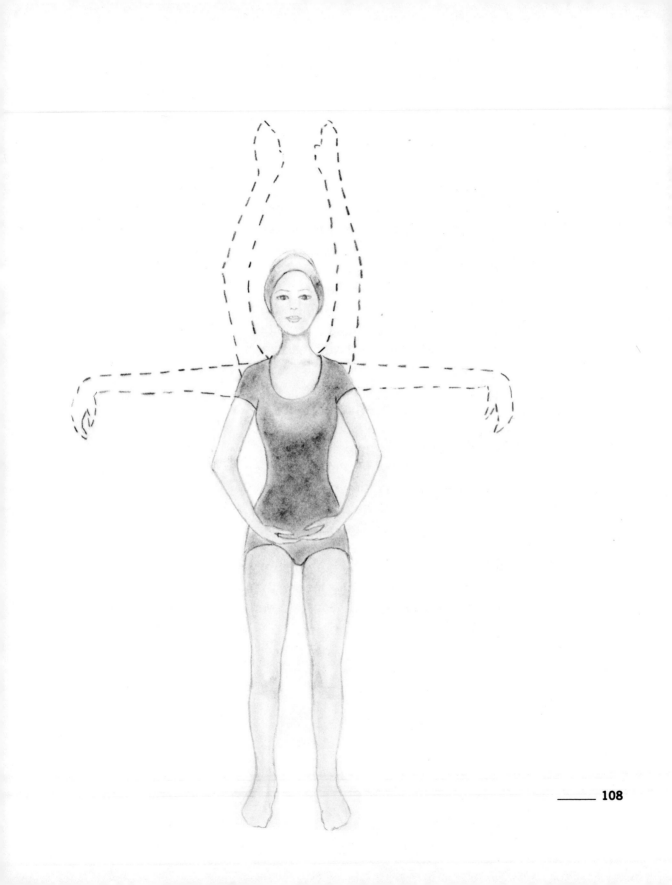

Standing Stretch

Stand erect. Exhale through mouth before breathing and stretching. Feet/legs together tight—knees straight.

With elbows slightly bent, place hands palms up and fingertips together in front of the base of the stomach. Slowly raise arms straight over the head while simultaneously inhaling (through the nose) at the same pace. Fill lungs to full capacity in this position.

With raised palms inward, elbows straight, knees straight, stretch, tighten the whole body and hold to the count of five.

Turn palms outward. Slowly exhale through the mouth, returning your arms to the sides with the palms pushing outward (fingertips up) on descent.

Hold position, exhale farther, pull up and tighten stomach muscles. Count five. Breathe normally. Repeat two times.

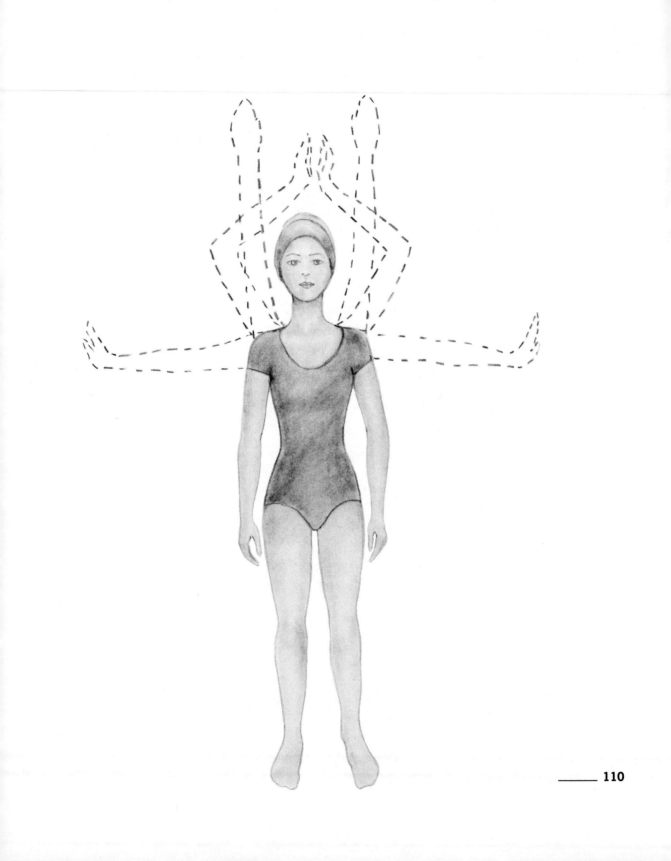

Pagoda Stretch

Stand erect, feet and legs together tight, knees straight. Arms by the sides (palms inward), elbows straight.

With elbows slightly bent, place hands parallel, palms up and fingertips together in front of the base of the stomach.

Slowly raise arms straight over the head while simultaneously inhaling through the nose at the same pace to the count of five. Fill lungs to full capacity in this position.

With raised palms inward, press them together, elbows slightly curved and parallel with the ears. Slowly lower the pressed palms with the wrist settling on the top of your head. Exhale slowly as you are lowering your palms and remember to keep your head erect. When you have let all breath out, inhale slowly to the same pace as you again raise your pressed palms to the stretch position.

Turn the palms outward, slowly exhale through the mouth, returning your arms to the sides with the palms pushing outward, fingertips up, on descent.

Hold, tighten stomach muscles ... count five. Repeat two times.

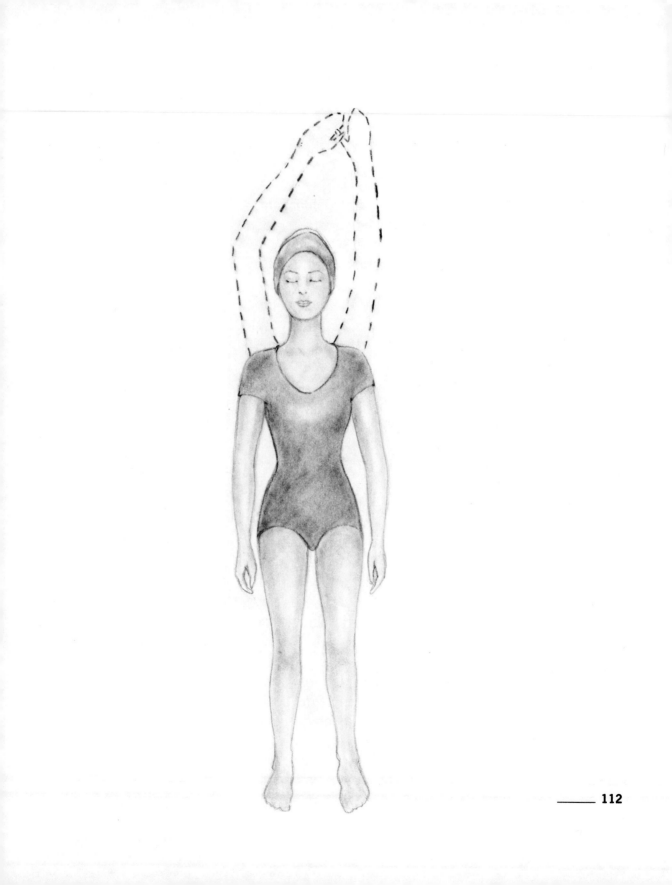

Thumb Stretch

Get into the same position of preparation as for the Standing Stretch. This time, with the arms raised to full stretch, grasp the right thumb with the left thumb and index finger and pull upward. Now grasp the left thumb with the right thumb and index finger and pull upward. You should be breathing in as your arms are raised and at the same pace. Exhale, lowering your arms slowly, to the count of five. Tighten stomach muscles. Repeat two times.

You will feel taller, alert and calm after these exercises. Do them every day.

······
THE BATH

*There's no place like a
bath to stretch your
soul and listen to your
inner voice.*
—Seneca

Your METAMASSAGE bathing technique will not take any longer than your
former bathing method if you apply
yourself. Read the instructions and observe the illustrations before taking your
bath or shower. Familiarize yourself
with the brushing motions and the
counting rules thoroughly. In a short
time both will become automatic, but
you must make the initial effort. No
one can make you do anything you
don't *want* to do. My purpose is not
only to help you look and feel better
by retarding the aging process, but to
inspire you to want to accomplish these
goals.

Your body is in the process of continually renewing its cell structure. Help
it by sloughing away the dead cells that
accumulate. This particular kind of
bath is the kindest thing that you can
do to assist your skin in its natural
function. The necessity of the brush

that you'll be using is to facilitate the removal of dead cells from the surface of the skin.

Since you reside in your body, begin to live by listening as your body talks to you in a language all its own. It tells you when and what to eat, when you need exercise and when to rest, when to move alone or with someone, and how to move, with an inordinate amount of freedom that you've never known. Your body movements while making love will be less restricted, and no part of you should be inaccessible. Why should it be? You're on the road to discovery!

Try to make your METAMASSAGE body habits part of the new, "routined" you. Your spirit will soar with your attitude of continuous refinement.

What You Need

For starters, a good, stiff (I said *stiff*) long-handled brush as fully bristled as you can find is a necessity. A natural bristle brush is preferable, but if you can't find a good one, Fuller Brush

Company makes an excellent nylon-bristled one.

For those of you who feel that a tub is only collecting dirty water around you, don't forget to use a water softener. If you're not fortunate enough to live in a community with soft water, try

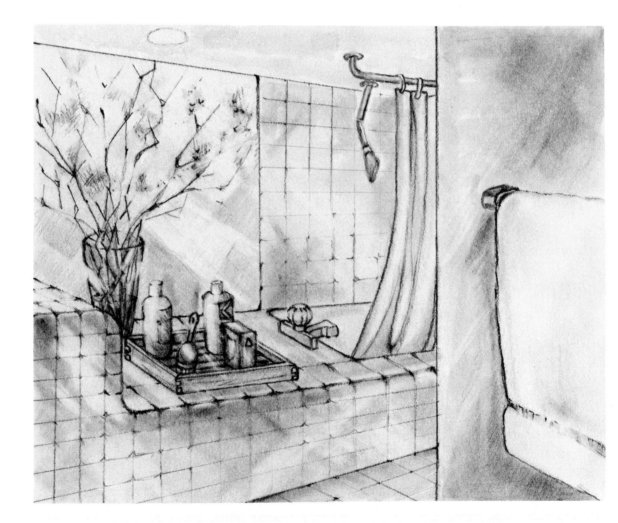

one of the commercial additives, such as Calgon water softener. You will find other suggestions in the SPA FOR-MULAS section.

You'll also need, of course, your favorite soap, preferably one that lathers easily. I switch brands constantly and will only recommend that you use the one you like best.

Get a big bottle of moisturizing body lotion (not oil), to moisturize your entire body when through.

A well-tufted bath towel or full-length terry cloth robe is necessary to absorb the excess water after you've completed your bath.

Be sure you have everything you'll need *before* you get started, and it will be a much more relaxing, pleasant experience. There's nothing worse than getting out of the tub with silky, smooth skin and no moisturizer on hand to help keep it that way!

Directions on both the brushing motions and the proper counting for each area of the body are made explicit with the accompanying illustrations. With brush in hand read them while looking at figures 14 through 23. Remember the count where stated.

If you do not have access to a tub and must shower, then the process of using the bath brush and counting is the same. While in the tub you have the advantage of immersion; in the shower you can relieve tension by allowing the water to run briskly over your body after completing the scrubbing. Use varying degrees of temperature, never too hot or too cold. A good practice is to combine the bath and shower routine. If at all possible, however, the bath should be used no less than four times a week.

THE ORDER OF YOUR BATH

1. Relax 5 minutes
2. Hands, wrist and elbows
3. Arms
4. Breasts and chest area
5. Shoulders, upper portion of back and nape of neck
6. Back and rib cage
7. Undercurve of arm and armpits
8. Stomach
9. Buttocks
10. Hip, upper and lower thighs
11. Knees, legs and feet
12. Relax, drain water
    RINSE

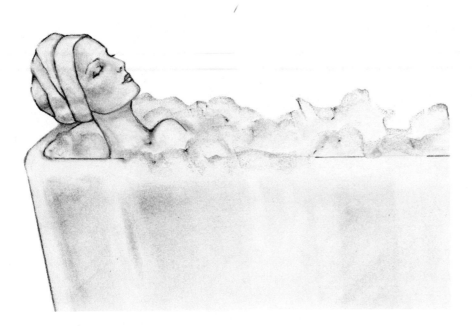

Figure 13 Prepare a bath with your favorite formula. When the tub is three-quarters full, slip into your luxurious suds and lie there for 5 minutes. Relax your body through conscious thought (actually tell your body, part by part, to relax). Begin with the toes and work up to the ends of the hair. This is a quiet time for yourself. Dream, but don't plan.

If taking a shower, begin by standing straight with your chin raised and let a light mist of water ripple from your cheeks over your whole body. Slowly turn with your back to the shower head. With your head relaxed forward, shut your eyes for a moment and think only of the water cascading down your body.

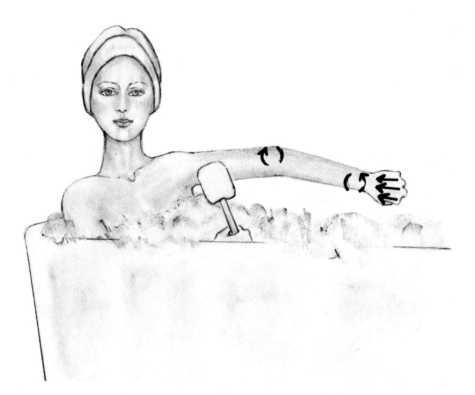

Figure 14 After your moments of relaxation, sit up and continue your routine by soaping the bath brush. Start with the hands and wrists. (I suggest the hands first because they are one of the most neglected parts of the body). With straight and circular brushing motions count twenty-five times just on this area.

When you have finished both hands, brush in a circular motion twenty-five times on first one elbow and then the other. The second most deprived area is the elbows. I start from right to left because I am right handed, but you should follow your instinctive preference so that you develop a routine you will not forget. (Remember, fifty times on one elbow will not, by osmosis, smooth the other. It is important to concentrate on what you are doing.)

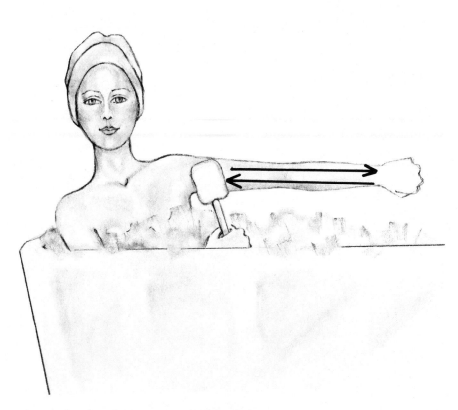

Figure 15 When you have finished the elbows, do the whole arms, fifteen strokes, working up and down on each arm. Remember that you go both up and down to complete one entire brush stroke.

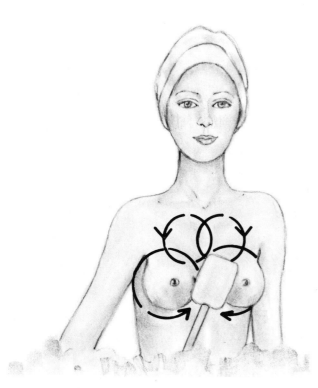

Figure 16 Still seated, rinse and resoap the brush after each series, or as often as necessary. Now, do at least fifteen motions around each breast, and do another fifteen directly above each breast on the chest. Be sure to overlap with the circular motions so that you do not cheat any portion of the breast and chest area. It is not necessary to go over the nipple with the brush as this would probably be irritating. You'll find that as you circle each breast the nipple and surrounding area will get enough soap to clean it.

Figure 17 With your bath brush you can easily reach all portions of the shoulders and upper back. Brush fifteen times on each shoulder and upper part of the back. Overlap toward the nape of the neck with your strokes.

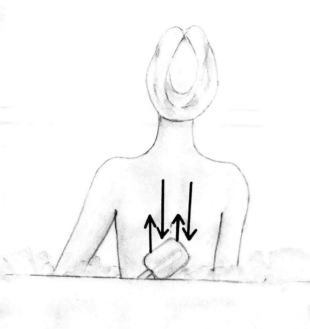

Figure 18 Rinse and resoap the brush and proceed to the lower portion of the back and rib cage area. Do a minimum of ten strokes on each side of the spine, being sure to overlap. Then do the same motions on the front of your body, starting from under the breasts and going down to the waistline. Brush between the breasts as well. There should be a minimum of ten strokes up and down on each of these torso areas.

Slide down into the water to rinse off all the soap. You will immediately feel glowingly warm and alive. Don't be afraid if the stiff bristles of your brush make your skin feel a bit tender and tingly. Soon you will not wish to bathe without your brush.

NOW SLOWLY STAND UP.

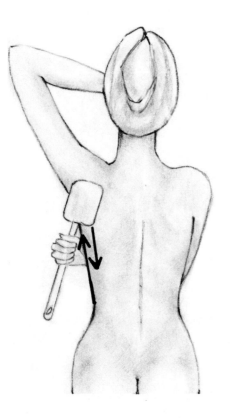

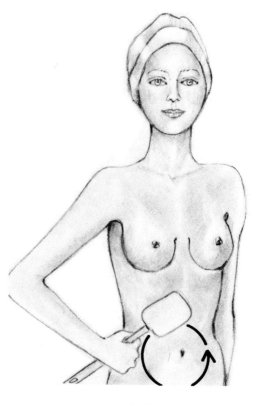

Figure 19 We are going to attend to another of those neglected areas, the undercurve of the arm on either side of the armpit. Do ten strokes on each side and gently stroke the armpit itself five or six times.

Figure 20 Still standing, rub your hand over your stomach to "desensitize" this delicate portion of the skin. Begin your ten count in a circular motion with a freshly soaped brush. (Truly, with many dunkings and resoapings of the brush it shouldn't be too inflexible by now.)

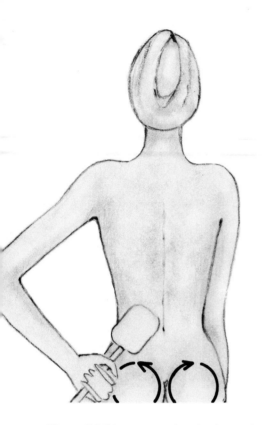

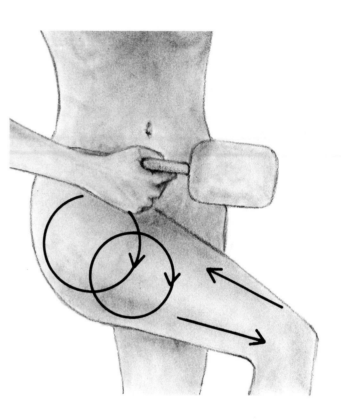

Figure 21 Move around to the buttocks, doing first ten motions on the left and then ten on the right... or more depending on whether the texture of the skin is rough or smooth. (You can, of course, reverse the order of left side to right side if it seems more natural to you.) Keep the motions circular.

Figure 22 Continue with ten to fifteen (again depending on the texture of your skin and how conscientiously you wish to smooth it) circular motions on the upper thighs, on each side. Then do ten to fifteen times just above that area on the hip. Next, do the same amount of strokes *up and down* and all around the thighs to the knee, on each leg.

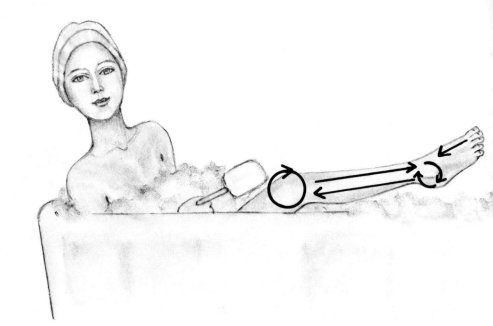

SLOWLY SIT DOWN AND SLIDE INTO THE WATER, RINSING THE SOAP OFF THE LOWER PART OF THE BODY.

Note: On the genital and anal areas, merely soap with your hand, or use a washcloth, taking care to rinse well.

If you work steadily and briskly over each portion of the body, it will not be necessary to rinse away the soap each time you cover an area however, you can scoop a handful of water over the area just brushed if you have dry skin.

Figure 23 With your foot up on the front rim of the tub, or in a bent position, brush fifteen circular motions on each knee. Then, from the knees to the ankles, do the same amount of strokes brushing up and down. The fifteen strokes include the back, front and sides of the leg.

On the feet, do ten strokes upward from the toes to the ankles. A few circular motions over and around the ankles feel wonderful.

Don't forget the soles and the heels but be gentle if you're ticklish!

Gently go around the cuticles on your hand and toe nails with an orange stick or your thumb nail to loosen them while your skin is softening in the water. Then pass lightly over them with the brush to remove any loose skin. Use a pumice stone on softened calluses. Circular motions are most effective.

IF YOU SHAVE YOUR LEGS AND UNDER-ARMS, this is the time to do it. With the water additives the tiny hairs will not float to the outer ring of your tub, but will gently sink to the bottom. *NOW IS THE TIME TO WASH YOUR HAIR IF YOU HAD PLANNED TO DO IT DURING YOUR BATH OR SHOWER.*

You are ready for the final step of your bath! If you washed your hair, rinse well and apply your conditioner or rinse. Pull the plug, lie back full length and let your troubles, cares, stiffness, tension and soap flow down the drain, taking your tiredness along with it all.

If you shower, again let the water cascade over your body, front, sides and back. Graduate the temperature of the water from warm to as cold as you can comfortably stand it. Perhaps you have the kind of shower head that gives a variety of nozzle changes and varying water pressure. If so, increase then decrease the force along with the changes of water temperature.

Rinse

Suppose you have washed and conditioned your hair. Remove the conditioner or rinse at the same time you splash water over your body. The best thing, of course, is to have a shower or hand nozzle that attaches to the faucet in your tub. Without either of these conveniences I use a cooking pan and happily pour water over my head and body. This is a good time to apply one of the special rinses mentioned in the section on HAIR. First sitting, then standing, cover yourself with water, varying the temperature, and rinse well.

At the end of your rinse session, run cold water over the hands and wrists and douse your feet and ankles several times with only cold water. The whole body will feel invigorated!

What You Need to Remember

1. Rinse and resoap your bath brush whenever necessary.

2. On which side you began each series so that you never miss or neglect one area.
3. Brush with the proper motions—and count.
4. After your bath or shower, rinse the brush with cold water and shake briskly. You'll want it fresh and stiff for your next bath.
5. Concentrate on what you're doing, not missing any parts of the body or cheating on the number of strokes.

After the Bath

Step carefully out of the tub or shower and wrap a large towel around your entire body, or step into a full length terry cloth robe if you have one. Don't dry yourself but remain wrapped in your cocoon, maintaining the moisture still on your body. Relax for a moment, letting the terry cloth absorb some of the wetness.

While you are still slick and soft (not quite fully dry) drop the towel or robe to your waist. Begin with the upper part and spread scads of body cream, rubbing well into the skin, over your arms, back, chest and rib cage to the waist. After completing the upper part of the body remove the towel or robe and massage the rest of your skin with the cream. Don't neglect the feet but do be sure there is no excess cream or moisture left before putting on your hose or shoes.

Once a week, carefully trim any excess cuticle from both the finger and toenails. Cut as little as possible then rinse with rubbing alcohol. A good, medicated foot powder is an excellent idea for feet in closed shoes or boots. Not only does it eliminate foot odor, it helps prevent any problems related to athlete's foot or fungus infections.

Continue rubbing the cream on the entire body until there is no excess. Keep your arms limber and try not to miss any of the skin on your back. Backs can be beautiful, too.

Although this self-massage may not be as luxurious as that given by a professional, remember that you are putting energy back into your body from your own hands. This is again what I mean by ENERGY REPLACEMENT THERAPY. You, helping yourself. The complete theory of METAMASSAGE is based on this concept. Allow some time to do for yourself. What others cannot do for you.

Your body is *you*, your constantly moving vehicle. Care for it, love it and hold yourself in great esteem. Soon you'll observe how people will look for any excuse just to touch your beautiful skin.

Special Therapeutic Baths

Sea Salt and Soda Bath

The heavily polluted atmosphere, earth and food filled with chemicals and acid rains are significant signs of our times. We all have a degree of radiation and metals in our systems. The cockroach, rat and shark have survived from prehistoric times because they have the ability to adapt to changing factors around them. There are many things we humans can do to compensate for our variable environment. One step we can take is the *Sea Salt and Soda Bath* which Frank Tingue, an incredible Los Angeles physiotherapist, told me was first devised by the U.S. Army following World War II.

After the atomic bomb was dropped in Japan, radiation from the blast was carried through the atmosphere for hundreds of miles. People on the island of Iwo Jima, 660 nautical miles south of Japan, were exposed to atomic ions as were all those in fringe areas of Nagasaki and Hiroshima, where the bombs were dropped.

Ions from radiation produce a similar reaction to people who come in contact with radiation in nuclear plants, X-ray technicians and to a lesser degree those who live in areas highly polluted from a number of sources. One is hard put to find a place on our lovely planet where the food, soil or air is not contaminated with radioactivity or poisonous chemicals. The *Sea Salt and Soda Bath*, used originally by the people of Iwo Jima, counteracts the atomic ions.

The more you come into contact with impurities the more often you should do the *Sea Salt and Soda Bath*. Once or twice a week, depending on the area in which you live or work, or every two weeks if you live in a relatively safe environment, take the time for this healthful bath. From the first immersion you will feel an increase in energy and more enthusiasm for living as you rid yourself of the pernicious substances with which we are assaulted every day.

Place one pound of sea salt and one pound of bicarbonate of soda in a three-quarters-full tub of water as hot as you can stand it. Slosh the water to completely dissolve the salt and soda.

Lie back and relax for a minimum of one-half to three-quarters of an hour. Try listening to music (although you should be careful not to put an electrical appliance close to the tub), read or do the full body relaxation technique. Drain the water but *DO NOT RINSE*. Blot your skin dry with a towel and go to bed. Take a bath or shower, as usual, the next morning.

You must use *sea salt* which can be purchased in a health food store or your local market. If you cannot find the salt in bulk, call a wholesale house that deals with organic products. Four-pound boxes of bicarbonate of soda are available in most supermarkets.

I promise you will feel one hundred percent better with your *Sea Salt and Soda Baths.*

Cool Wash Scrub

My yoga teacher, with whom I studied for twenty-two years and who encouraged me to develop the METAMASSAGE technique, suggested the following stimulating procedure. Once or twice a week take a semi-cold shower without using soap, but briskly scrubbing with a water-softened bath brush or loofah. Then vigorously rub dry with a well-tufted bath towel. Use a body splash after this spartan regimen, and glow...

Spa at Home

Thy baths shall be the juice of July flowers, spirit of roses and violets, the milk of unicorns and panther's breath, gathered in bags and mixed with wines.

—Ben Jonson

Throughout history man has sought a fountain of youth. There are mineral hot springs all over the world in which man from the Pleistocene Epoch until today has relieved his aching body. Not only is it therapeutic to soak in these waters, the healing powers carry mystical overtones. For this reason the Romans revered the baths and also considered them a social event, while the Japanese continue this practice. Communal bathing has regained its popularity elsewhere, especially with the advent of the hot tub. Your *Spa at Home* will so excite you with its therapeutic powers you'll want to tell everyone to try it!

Soaking softens the skin so that when you use a bath brush you can easily slough off the dead cells that work their way to the surface of the skin (or epidermis) approximately every two weeks. Immersion in warm water is not only relaxing but healing. Rough skin, goose-bumped thighs, buttocks and arms; flab and stretch marks will diminish appreciably as you continue to METAMASSAGE your way to beautiful and silky, smooth skin.

DO NOT ADD THE OILS TO YOUR BATH UNTIL AFTER THE FIVE TO TEN MINUTE SOAK, BEFORE STARTING YOUR BATH ROUTINE. They are most effective when the skin is softened and the pores are open.
POUR IN DELICIOUS-SMELLING ROSE OR ORANGE FLOWER WATER FOR A REAL TREAT.

FLOAT IN:

Petals of roses, violets, gardenia or goldenrod... Scoop out before draining bath water.

Put the flowers or herbs in four thicknesses of cheesecloth and boil in two quarts of water. Add the water to your bath. Use the herbs to improve the skin if you bathe in the morning; to ease aches before going to bed in the evening; to soothe and calm in the morning or as a combination with the other herbs in the evening. You may also use tea bags in whichever herbs

SPA FORMULAS:

Pour In

BASIC BATH FORMULA

SOFTENERS—	Calgon Apple Cider Vinegar Cornstarch Bicarbonate of Soda	1 cup of each or any combination that suits you

*BUBBLERS AND
    THERAPEUTIC—*
	"Batherapy"
	"Olbas"
	"Vitabath"
	"Badedas"
	"Milk Bath,"
	    or
	    Your Favorite
		1 capful or according to direction

FUN ADDITIVES

Slice In

Lemon Slices
Orange and Lemon Peel

Drop in oils
(ten to fifteen drops only)

Wheat Germ Olive Avocado Sunflower Sesame Safflower Clove Patchouli Almond	Pine Oil for Congestion or Respiratory Problems Eucalyptus for Colds or Sinus Obstruction

More Spa Formulas

Herbs

To Improve Skin	To Ease Aches	To Soothe and Calm
Ginseng	Bay	Peppermint
Comfrey	Nutmeg	Camomile
Lemon Verbena	Oregano	Valerian Root
Cloves	Hayflower	Thyme
Goldenrod	Wintergreen	Passion Flower
St. Johns Wort	Purple or Yellow Iris	Hops
Red Raspberry	Deadly Nightshade	Tiger Lily
Foxglove	Dandelion	Lady's Slipper
Juniper	Grape Leaves	Peony

or flowers that are available. Typically a large variety of herbs can be found in health food stores or from an herbalist—these formulas are so relaxing that it's well worth the trouble of finding them!

Seaweed

Although it's not yet well known in America, in many parts of the world a seaweed soak is used for relaxation and balancing the system for weight loss. Oriental thought teaches that sea-weed stimulates the endocrine and lymphatic systems. Inga Schiller, a physiotherapist trained in Germany and now living in California, worked in spas in Europe where they used the following procedure: Prepare the packaged seaweed in the same manner as you do the herbs. Add three or four cups of sea salt to the bath water if you take the seaweed bath in the mornings, as it will be more stimulating. If you take the bath in the evening eliminate the sea salt for greater relaxation. Soak in the seaweed bath twenty minutes a day for one month in order to help weight loss.

**LAVENDER LEAVES* steeped in boiled water (use the same method as with rosemary leaves, wrapping them in cheesecloth) and added to the bath with any of the above combinations removes body odor. Add both the water and the bag of leaves to your bath, squeezing the excess water out first to get the true essence.

External Douche

Unfortunately, very few homes outside of Western Europe have a bidet in the bathroom. Nothing is more convenient than this relatively unavailable fixture to clean the perineal or genital area of the body. The sitting position on the bidet is perfect for a method of external douching hundreds of years old. In lieu of a bidet, this cleansing can be done in a squatting position near water or semi-reclining in a bathtub.

Since the greater part of vaginal secretions are in the lower section of the vaginal cavity one can cleanse this area without inserting nozzles or tubes. Depending if you are left or right handed, place the index, middle and ring fingers approximately one inch into the vaginal opening. Relax the muscles and gently press the backs of the fingers against the vaginal wall. With your other hand pour or splash water into the cupped hand still in the vagina. Press the fingers back against the wall each time you pour water into the cupped hand. Do this several times, then with one or two fingers clean around the muscular pockets just inside the opening. Don't be afraid to touch your body! Use as much water as is necessary. Having completed this portion of the douche, soap your hand and wash thoroughly the perineal or outside area. Rinse well.

Most doctors prefer that a woman not douche regularly except if, for example, she is using a cream or a diaphragm as a form of contraception. The *External Douche* does not present the same problems as an internal one. Your hands will be clean and you are not putting a bacteria-laden foreign object inside your body. When cleaning the genital area, however, make sure not to get soap in the vagina, as it can irritate the delicate tissues.

Around the anal area I use the bath brush if in the bath or shower. If I wish to clean the genitalia without bathing or showering, I make sure to use different hands for the anal and vaginal areas. Let me remind you to always wash your hands first.

Important Note: Wash and resoap the brush *before* and *after* you use it in the anal area. The spread of bacteria from the rectum can produce an infection in the vaginal or the urinary hollow. Remember what your gynecologist told you about wiping from back to front after a bowel movement. Don't do it!

METAMASSAGE AS A LIFETIME DISCIPLINE

One has to think of oneself differently. To change the picture you have of yourself, you must first *want* to change it. For some this takes more effort than for others. The secret is *discipline*.

Acknowledge a philosophy which motivates your activities. Investigate why you are doing what. If you're not happy with your mental attitude, skin or body, do something about it. Don't vent your frustrations and feelings of shortcoming on everyone around you.

Care about yourself and others will care about you. Take time for yourself and you will have time for everyone else. What better moment to start than at this or any juncture of your life while setting your future patterns of discipleship.

Do METAMASSAGE exactly as suggested throughout this book and don't neglect THE MORNING AFTER, following the facial routine. The results come so fast when it is done correctly that many people reach a plateau of satisfaction and stop. But when you stop, the improvement stops. Discipline is a way of life. It is also the only way to achieve anything, whether it be personal or professional.

If you have been doing METAMASSAGE religiously but you miss the routine one night, do a session the next morning, even if it's only twenty-five times each place for the three series. Do the same cleansing routine, then use:

Water around the eyes, astringent on the rest of the face and the neck, and put moisturizer on the neck and eye areas as shown in the illustrations. Follow the moisturizer with a bit of tepid water on cotton. This will take away any over-shine. On the neck, simply use enough cream so that you don't pull the skin. Repeat the water process if necessary. Pat dry cornstarch on the remainder of the face with cotton and leave it on for five to ten minutes. Gently whisk it off. Your skin will not feel greasy but smooth and firm.

Be sure to take good care of your hands and feet. The extremities are especially important because they reveal how much you really care about your whole body. Take the time to use a clear nail varnish on the nails of both feet and hands. If you prefer, color them. Be sure to change polish, even the clear enamel, if it is chipped or peeling. Through METAMASSAGE your cuticles should be in good shape. Go on, put a little extra hand cream on them as well. Don't neglect the stretch-breathing or bathing routine either.

It is never too early to begin total body care. You're at an exciting time in your life. Get in tune with yourself and use your new techniques and knowledge. Don't sulk; METAMAS-SAGE.

OTHER THINGS I DO

I only do facial exercises after META-MASSAGING my face and while the cream is still on, otherwise the skin is stretched unnecessarily.

I use a mask before going out whenever I wish to feel special.

To minimize the lines from the corner of the nostrils to the corners of the mouth I do the following exercise: with the lips closed but not pursed, force air into the upper lip region by pushing upward with the bottom lip. Release the air by gently blowing out. Repeat the exercise twenty times. When METAMASSAGING my face, I keep the upper lip ballooned and do tiny circular motions twenty-five times up and down the nose to mouth corridor before releasing the air gradually.

I have a grudge against gravity! At least once and whenever possible twice or three times a day I lie on a slant board for thirty minutes each time. This helps the flow of blood to the brain and places the bodily organs in proper alignment. This is particularly effective for the skin after doing your META-MASSAGE as it increases circulation. I try not to let gravity get me down!

When I feel lethargic or depressed I massage my face and neck with the "Meta" method or I take "the" bath. Many times I do both, as it always gives me a lift.

If even a tiny line anywhere in the eye area tries to sneak in, I do fifty to one hundred extra tiny circular motions (gently) on the line when META-MASSAGING my face and neck. Actually extra circular motions any place where you see lines encroaching lessen them almost immediately. Repeat the practice two or three days running or until the line fades to your satisfaction.

I constantly remind myself not to squint, frown or stretch the skin by resting my face in my hands.

Bodies repair themselves when they rest or sleep. I make sure I have extra time to relax as much as I can when tired or playing hard.

I do an extra session of facial META-MASSAGE in the morning whenever I miss a night of the routine.

I continue to discipline myself to count whether cleansing my face or body, also when exercising or doing breathing exercises.

I organize my time. I have all the time and freedom in the world as long as I take care of the important things first.

I watch my diet and try not to over-eat.

Occasionally I switch all of the products I use on my face or body and experiment with new ones on the market.

I use toothpicks, Stimudents, dental floss, a Water Pik, and brush my teeth with disciplined regularity. Twice a week I use a combination of one-half bicarbonate of soda and sea salt to clean my teeth and mouth.

When I bend down to retrieve a

dropped object I exhale completely then pull up my stomach muscles and rise slowly. I learned that by keeping the sternum up I have more control over my body, breathe more deeply and stand tall.

I try to make exercise a continuing stream of consciousness by maintaining good posture.

I make every attempt not to over-extend myself by placating others. I save energy by being able to say no, if necessary.

When at a social function I repair to the closest plumbing at the moment of need. After washing my hands and before drying them, I gently pat my face and neck and let it dry, then press powder on my forehead, nose and chin. If my eyes are lined with pencil I reline them and touch up the mascara. With a few brush or finger strokes on the hair and a fresh application of lipstick or gloss, no matter how tired I am, I appear vital and fresh. This really works, gang, and only takes five minutes or less!

I regularly give myself a manicure and pedicure.

I take vitamins, minerals, herbs and cell salts according to what my body tells me it needs.

I sleep well because I refuse to carry each day's vicissitudes into the state of slumber. I don't wish to muddy another dimension of life in which I can dream away frustration or explore my fantasies.

I maintain a sense of humor about myself and life in general. I try to be tolerant, understanding and non-judgmental. Life is a never ending stream of trial and error, and nobody is perfect!

CARE ENOUGH

Let me emphasize once again the importance of taking the time to care for yourself. Whether you do this technique every night or three times a week, *do it*. Each session makes a visible difference. And when you do it, do it correctly and do it well. In a very short time you will have the technique down pat. It is *within you* to change your inner as well as your outer self. *Now* is the time to change your total attitude about yourself. *Now* means it's never too late to begin, whether you're a teenager struggling for a blemish-free complexion, or a woman who is concerned about the tiny lines beginning to appear around her eyes.

Youth itself is an attitude. My mother is seventy-eight and rarely misses doing METAMASSAGE. She was in intensive care for a heart condition for five days. When she came home from the hospital she took a good look at herself in the mirror. She had lain in the hospital in misery not knowing where the mystery of life was taking her. It was not so much the balance between life and death that weakened her, but the feeling of helplessness and impotency that comes from being ill.

Mother's first comment after turning from the mirror was that she had never thought she looked old before. She promptly got into bed, propped herself against some pillows and METAMESSAGED. Immediately her color returned. As her feelings of regeneration returned through her own store of energy, her attitude about herself began to change. Within two days she

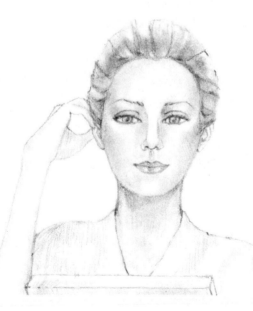

felt and looked her beautiful self again. Not one thing, but many different things are the panacea of life.

At 53 my life has taken up where it left off during those child-rearing years. Now that my children are grown I have begun again my career where I chose to desert it. The world has not passed me by, nor am I middle-aged, lonely or lacking in self-confidence. I feel good about myself...no tell-tale lines or heavy drooping jowls make me hesitate for one moment to face each day with renewed enthusiasm. The time I have spent on myself is as precious as any that has been given to my loved ones. We have not been in competition for time spent—they are important, but so am I! I have learned to take care of myself and so must you—no one's going to do it for you. For me META-MASSAGE has been a survival technique for looking good, feeling good about myself and remaining young in body and spirit. It's worked for me and countless others who have learned my technique, and it'll work for you!

Youth is not a time of life—it is a state of mind, a temper of the will, a quality of the imagination, a vigor of the emotions, a freshness of the deep springs of life. Nobody grows old merely by living a number of years; people grow old by deserting their ideals. Years wrinkle the skin but to give up enthusiasm wrinkles the soul. Whether sixty or sixteen, there is in every human heart the lure of wonder, the undaunted challenge of events, the unfailing childlike appetite for what's next, and the joy of the game of living. We are as young as our self-confidence, as old as our fear; as young as our desire, as old as our despair.

—Anonymous

Bibliography

Gray's Anatomy. Warren H. Lewis.

Standard Textbook of Cosmetology, rev. ed. Constance V. Kibbe, 1981. Milady Publishing Co.

Infant and Child in the Culture of Today: The Guidance of Development in Home and Nursery School. rev. ed. Arnold Gesell et al. 1974. Harper and Row.

Phenomenon of Man. Pierre Teilhard De Chardin. Harper & Row.

East-West Journal. East-West Cultural Institute. Boston, Mass.

Dr. Zizmor's Skin Care Book. Jonathan Zizmor, M.D., and John Foreman. 1977. Holt, Rinehart and Winston.

Let's Eat Right to Keep Fit, rev. ed. Adele Davis. 1970. Harcourt, Brace and Jovanovich.

Slanting Board. Bernard Jensen. Bernard Jensen Products, Solana Beach, Ca. 92075.